GROWING MARIJUANA

A Quick Start Indoor/Outdoor Grower's Guide for Medical and Personal Marijuana Cultivation

G Keller & R. Moore

Table of Contents

Introduction

Marijuana faced a long period of prohibition in the United States, as well as in some other countries around the world. In the past couple decades, however, the attitude toward marijuana has shifted. Select states have even gone as far as legalizing cannabis, either for medical or recreational use. In some areas, it is even legal to grow your own cannabis and sell it to the state for profit if you have the right paperwork.

In this book, you will learn everything that you need to know to grow marijuana. This will cover steps for indoor and outdoor growing, how to legally grow in your area, tips for choosing where to grow and average costs, tips for troubleshooting your cannabis crop if you have pest or mold growth, how to cure your harvest when it reaches maturity, and more.

You will find that this all-inclusive guide is broken into sections labeled as steps. Within these individual steps, you will find that there are one or more chapters. The reason for this is that there are different methods for growing marijuana. You will find information for growing indoors or outdoors from a seed or a clone, as well as different techniques and set-ups for your marijuana operation. To help you locate the specific information for your growing method, you will be able to skip directly to the chapters that you need.

Thank you for reading this book and happy growing!

Step 1: Growing Legally in Your Area

Chapter 1: The History and Prohibition of Cannabis and Marijuana in the United States

Marijuana has a long history of prohibition in the United States, starting with cannabis. It was introduced as early as the 17th century, when hemp was encouraged for use in clothing, sales, and more. Many centuries later, its recreational usage was noticed and propaganda had many groups speaking out against it. Marijuana has a long and rich history in the United States- read on to learn more.

Earliest Known Use in the United States

Cannabis first caught the attention of settlers in the early 1600s, when the American government realized its many benefits for production. They encouraged farmers to produce hemp and it was used for production of clothing, sails, rope, and other useful cloth items. In the year 1619, recommendation became requirement as the Virginia Assembly legislated a law that required every farmer living in the area to grow hemp. This was quite advantageous to them and spurred the wealth of small farmers, because hemp could be used as legal tender in Virginia, Pennsylvania, and Maryland.

The end of the Civil War saw the end of the era where hemp was so popular. Domestic materials and imports started to replace the hemp for many production purposes.

Around the same time, medicinal doctors and herbalists took note of the cannabis plant for another reason- its medicinal properties. It was not uncommon for over-the-counter products to include this now popular ingredient that could be sold legally in public pharmacies.

Recreationally, marijuana was not very common during this time. A byproduct of marijuana called hashish did, however, become popular around the 19th century. It was especially popular in France but eventually spread to some areas of the United States.

First Labeling of Marijuana

In the year 1906, the United States government passed its first federal regulation concerning marijuana. This small piece of legislation called the Pure Food and Drug Act required that any supplements containing any form of marijuana or the cannabis plant be labeled.

The Mexican Revolution and How it Brought Marijuana to the United States

While hashish was smoked in some areas, marijuana

smoking was not popular in the United States in the first decade of the 1900s. In 1910, the Mexican Revolution started and brought with it widespread violence across Mexico in one of the most significant uprisings of the 20th century. In response to the intense violence across the country, many Mexican families immigrated to the United States. With them, they brought their recreational use of marijuana.

The Earliest Anti-Marijuana Campaigns

The use of marijuana by the new foreigners to the United States did not go over well, especially once anti-drug groups started to spread their propaganda. Since marijuana had been brought over with the Mexican immigrants, it was associated with the same fear and prejudice as foreigners were. It was this fear and prejudice that led to the propaganda of the time, which associated the "Marijuana Menace", as it was called, with Mexicans, poverty, lower class communities, and crime. This early prejudice would lead to the prejudiced research a few decades later.

The Great Depression and the Outlawing of Marijuana in the United States

The stock market crashed in 1929 and led to the Great Depression, which would be known as one of the most poverty-stricken decades in American history. This led to poverty across all communities but struck the lower class especially hard, as families that worked hard to just scrape by now had no way to pay for food, living quarters, and other amenities.

Massive unemployment across the country left nearly 3.2 million Americans out of work. Instead of placing the blame on the banks of Wall Street and major players that contributed to the stock market crash, the American people began to place blame on the Mexican immigrants. This new fear of immigrants and what they could do led to research of the recreational marijuana that had been brought over from their home country.

Of course, the studies of the time found that marijuana was linked to lower class communities such as immigrants and other minorities. In addition to linking marijuana with low-class use, the studies found it connected to crime, violence, and a whole slew of deviant behaviors. This led to the first legislation against marijuana use on a state level, with 29 states outlawing the use of the drug by the year 1931.

The Beginning of Federal Marijuana Prohibition

Individual states are responsible for setting their own legislation on marijuana. This is something that is true even today, though as you will see, this created issues between state and federal government when they disagreed.

The first steps toward federal prohibition began with the establishment of the Federal Bureau of Narcotics or FBN. This coincided with the appointment of Harry J. Anslinger as commissioner in 1930. He would go on to hold this position for 32 years.

Under him, the first marijuana prohibition was passed. The federal government did not want to be responsible for the enforcement of the marijuana laws of the time, so they permitted the individual states to set their own rules. They were heavily encouraged, however, to pass the Uniform State Narcotic Act. This act established a strong stand against the use of marijuana within each state's individual territory, a stand which each of the states adopted to outlaw marijuana across the United States.

More Marijuana Propaganda and the Banning of Narcotics in Film

From the mid-1930s to the mid-1940s, marijuana propaganda showed up everywhere. One of the most notable films was produced by Louis Gasnier, a French director. The film titled *Reefer Madness* was pushed on teens and their parents. It told the story of teens who had used marijuana and come under the inflection of a disease known as reefer madness.

The film was developed in an era where the decision to use marijuana was a moral choice. Those pushing anti-marijuana propaganda believed that it ruined the human spirit and turned teens and other users into fiends. They would enjoy the buzz but soon feel the need for more and would eventually make questionable decisions like stealing from their parents or robbing a bank to feed their addiction. Reefer madness could also affect young women, destroying their spirits and turning them into fools and whores. The only known cure for this affliction was a long period of sobriety from any type of alcohol or narcotics.

In addition to the propaganda of the time, the use of any narcotics (including marijuana) was banned in film. This was set forth by the Motion Pictures Association of America, which was made up of the major Hollywood studios of the time in 1936.

Complete Marijuana Prohibition: The Marijuana Tax Act of 1937

Following a very widespread campaign that reached all corners of the United States, the Marijuana Tax Act was passed by Congress in 1937. This was the first time that it was no longer up to the individual states and the federal government stepped in to ban marijuana. Marijuana was completely criminalized upon the passing of this statute and possession was restricted only to those who paid a luxury tax for authorized industrial or medical uses.

The First Steps Toward Legalization of Marijuana

In the 1940s, hemp and similar materials were necessary in large supply because of World War II. These types of materials were used to make parachutes, cordage, and other necessary equipment for the military and marines. This spurred an initiative called "Hemp for Victory", which was a farming program. Farmers participating in the program were provided cannabis seeds to grow hemp. In addition to the seeds they needed for planting, they were granted deferment from the military draft of the time. This led to an impressive 375,000 acres of total hemp grown by the year 1943.

Also during this time, in the year 1944, the La Guardia Report was published. This was the first report to contradict the studies of previous years, finding that there was no correlation between marijuana use and sex crimes, insanity, and violent acts. Additionally, the La Guardia Report found no relationship between the use of marijuana and the use of harder drugs, disproving claims that it was a "gateway" drug.

Increased Marijuana Prohibition

The findings of the La Guardia Report did not affect public opinion at all. The Boggs Act of 1952 and Narcotics Control Act of 1956 both made stricter mandatory sentencing laws for those caught in possession of or growing marijuana. Even someone found in possession of marijuana for the first time faced a minimum of 2 years in jail or as much as 10 years, accompanied by a fine up to $20,000.

Shifting Attitudes

In the 1960s, public opinion began to shift on the treatment of people found in possession of marijuana, in favor of a more lenient punishment and medical treatment over jail time. This could have been because of the shift of marijuana use from only lower class groups to the upper white middle class. Both President Kennedy and President Johnson instructed that reports be conducted on the use of marijuana. These reports agreed with the La Guardia Report, saying that marijuana did not cause deviant behavior and that it did not lead to heavier drug use.

In 1968, a more organized group for fighting the use of drugs for marijuana was created when the FBN and the Food and Drug Administration's Bureau of Dangerous Drugs were merged.

1970: A Milestone Year for the Lift of Marijuana Prohibition

As the studies were released and anti-marijuana propaganda slowly faded, Congress took note of the shift. It was also noted that the drug culture of the 1960's that embraced the use of cannabis was not influenced by the mandatory sentences established a decade earlier. The inability of these laws and the general feeling that they were unnecessarily harsh led to the repeal of most of the mandatory penalties of the previous decades.

Another step was taken when the Comprehensive Drug Abuse Prevention and Control Act was passed. This statute eliminated mandatory sentencing on a federal level for possession of marijuana in small amounts and categorized cannabis separately from the much more dangerous narcotics that it was grouped with before.

Finally, NORML was established. The National Organization for the Reform of Marijuana Laws is a lobbyist group in Washington. They are non-profit and have the main goal of legalizing marijuana throughout the entire country.

The Effects of the Findings of the Shaffer Committee

In 1972, Congress decided that further investigation was needed into public opinion of marijuana and its effects on communities. President Nixon followed their direction and appointed the Shaffer Committee. This committee reviewed the materials disproving the links between marijuana, hard drug use, and deviant behavior, as well as the current federal laws in place and public attitude toward these laws and marijuana use. The Shaffer Committee recommended that President Nixon take the necessary actions to decriminalize marijuana for personal use, however, he did not take their recommendations at the time. Their findings still were a factor in the decriminalization of marijuana in eleven different states throughout the 1970s. Those that chose not to decriminalize, for the most part, reduced penalties.

Other Notable Events in the 1970s

The US DEA or Drug Enforcement Agency was established in 1973. This was created by merging the Office of Drug Abuse Law Enforcement and the Bureau of Narcotics and Dangerous Drugs.
In 1974, High Times magazine was put into print. This was the first easily accessible literature available that promoted the use and legalization of cannabis.

The Next Roadblocks

While the decriminalization of marijuana in many states and the founding of High Times magazine marked huge milestones, the fight against marijuana prohibition was far from over. Parents began to lobby against marijuana once again in 1976. They were disgusted by the idea of their teens using the drug and many of the groups were quite effective in getting their message across. They worked with the National Institute on Drug Abuse and the DEA to spread propaganda and their message about the problems with teens using marijuana. The influence that they had eventually began to shift some public attitude toward marijuana and helped contribute to the War on Drugs of the 1980s.

A key event of the War on Drugs was the Anti-Drug Abuse Act. While most of the legislation of the previous decades had been slowly decriminalizing marijuana, this put forth harsher federal penalties for possession of marijuana, especially those caught dealing. This act was signed into effect in 1986 and it strengthened the ideas put forth by the Comprehensive Crime Control Act put into effect in 1984. Large amounts of marijuana were punishable based on the amounts found and someone found with 100 grams of heroin was punished the same as someone found with 100 marijuana plants. An amendment to this law established a more severe penalty, with life-long sentences being the penalty for someone found in possession of large amounts of drugs three times and death sentences allowed to be dealt out to the dealers at the top of the chain.

The New War on Drugs

During President's George H.W. Bush's reign in the White House, he declared a need for an all-new war on drugs. While the numbers of current drug users had declined significantly, there was a new epidemic in the forms of cocaine and heroin addiction. He believed that one of the keys to beating this was drug education that should be implemented early in the school years. He also stated that steps must be taken to stop teens from starting use of drugs early, even marijuana.

Finally: Legalization

Though there were federal laws in place prohibiting

marijuana sale at the time, Proposition 215 was passed in California in 1996. California became the first state to take steps toward legalization, though their legalization only applied to the medical sale and use of marijuana to patients with serious and painful conditions such as cancer or AIDS. The conflict between federal laws and state laws caused a struggle, but this still marked a major milestone toward marijuana legalization. As you will see in the next chapter, other states would follow.

Chapter 2: Current Marijuana Laws and Considerations for Legal Growing

Since the legalization of marijuana by California, more states have followed closely in their footsteps. Cannabis is regulated on the state level, so the rules that apply in some states do not apply in others. In this chapter, you will find all the states that currently have marijuana legalized on some level, as of June 2016. If you do not see your state here, do a little research of your own. Additionally, laws change with time, so be sure to check the most recent information even if your state is listed here to see if there have been any repeals or amendments!

Medical Marijuana Laws

This list covers the states that allow possession for medical consumption. Many even allow you to grow your own plants if you pay taxes on them and fill out the right paperwork. Be sure to check the specific regulations in your area before you decide to grow so that you can do so legally.

1. **California**- Proposition 215 passed with 56% of the vote in 1996. Small amounts are allowed in amounts up to 8 ounces and you can either possess 12 immature plants or 6 mature plants.

2. **Alaska**- Alaska approved Ballot Measure 8 with a 58% approval rating in 1998. It allows an individual to be in possession 1 ounce marijuana to be used for medical use and the ability to grow up to 6 plants, 3 of them mature and 3 of them immature.

3. **Washington**- In 1998, Initiative 692 passed with a 59% yes vote, legalizing possession of up to 24 ounces of medical marijuana and 15 plants.

4. **Oregon**- Ballot Measure 67 passed with a 55% approval rating in 1998. It allows possession of up to 24 ounces of dried marijuana and 24 total plants, with a maximum of 6 being in a mature stage.

5. **Maine**- Medical marijuana became legal in 1999 in Maine with a 61% yes vote on Ballot Question 2. Individuals can possess up to 2.5 ounces of bud and grow as many as 6 plants.

6. **Colorado**- In 2000, Ballot Amendment 20 passed with a 54% yes vote. This allows 2 ounces of marijuana to be in your possession and the ability to grow 3 mature plants and 3 immature plants.

7. **Hawaii**- Senate Bill 862 was passed in 2000 with a vote of 13-12 in the Senate and 32-18 in the House. It allows up to 4 ounces of cannabis to be in an individual's possession and up to 7 plants to be grown.

8. **Nevada**- The legalization of medical marijuana in Nevada happened in 2000, when Ballot Question 9 passed with a 65% approval rate. It allows patients to have 2.5 ounces of usable marijuana and as many as 12 plants.

9. **Montana**- Initiative 148 was approved with a 62% yes vote in 2004. It allows possession of 1 ounce of dried marijuana, 4 mature plants, and as many as 12 seedlings.

10. **Vermont**- In 2004, Senate Bill 76 passed with votes of 85-29 in the House and 22-7 in the Senate to legalize possession of medical marijuana in the amount of 2 ounces. It also allows growth of 9 plants; 2 mature and 7 immature.

11. **Rhode Island**- Senate Bill 0710 passed with votes of 33-1 in the Senate and 52-10 in the House. As of 2006, it allows possession of up to 2.5 ounces of marijuana and 12 plants.

12. **New Mexico**- Marijuana was legalized in 2007 with the passing of Senate Bill 523 with votes of 32-3 in the Senate and 36-31 in the House. It allows possession of 6 ounces of marijuana, 4 mature plants, and 12 immature plants.

13. **Michigan**- In 2008, Proposal 1 passed with a 63% approval rating to legalize possession of medical marijuana up to 2.5 ounces. Medical marijuana patients are also allowed to grow up to 12 plants.

14. **DC-** Washington DC legalized marijuana in 2010 with the passing of Amendment Act B18-622. This passed with a 13-0 vote and allows for 2 ounces of dried medical marijuana to be possessed, with the set limits on other types of marijuana byproducts to be decided later.

15. **Arizona-** Proposition 203 passed in 2010 with just over 50% of the vote. This permits someone to possess up to 2.5 ounces of marijuana and 12 plants.

16. **New Jersey-** The passing of Senate Bill 119 with 25-13 in the Senate and 48-14 in the House legalized marijuana in 2010 for New Jersey residents. It allows possession of 2 ounces of marijuana.

17. **Delaware-** The enactment of Senate Bill 17 legalized marijuana in Delaware with a vote of 27-14 in the House and 17-4 in the Senate. As of 2011, residents of Delaware with a medical marijuana license can possess up to 6 ounces of marijuana.

18. **Massachusetts-** Marijuana was legalized with a 63% vote for Ballot Question 3 in 2012. The possession limit is a 60-day supply, not to amount to more than 10 ounces.

19. **Connecticut-** Connecticut legalized marijuana in 2012 with the passing of House Bill 5389, which passed 21-13 in the Senate and 96-51 in the House. Possession of up to 2.5 ounces is legal for medical use.

20. **New Hampshire-** New Hampshire legalized medical marijuana with a voting of 18-6 in the Senate and

284-66 in the House on House Bill 573 in 2013. It allows possession of up to 2 ounces of cannabis for use of no less than a period of 10 days.

21. **Illinois**- House Bill 1 passed with a 35-21 vote in the Senate and a 61-57 vote in the House in 2013. This allows possession of 2.5 ounces of dried cannabis to be in your possession to be used over a minimum period of 14 days.

22. **Minnesota**- Senate Bill 2470 passed with an 89-40 vote in the House and a 46-16 vote in the Senate to legalize medical marijuana in Minnesota in 2014. It allows patients to be in possession of a 30-day supply of marijuana, though it must be in a non-smokeable form.

23. **New York**- New York legalized in 2014 with the passing of Assembly Bill 6357 with 49-10 in the Senate and 117-13 in the Assembly of Congress. It allows patients to possess a 30-day supply of marijuana in a non-smokeable form.

24. **Maryland**- In 2014, House Bill 881 passed with a vote of 44-2 in the Senate and 125-11 in the House to legalize medical marijuana possession of a supply for 30 days, with the acceptable amount to be set at some time in the future.

25. **Ohio**- House Bill 523 passed with votes of 71-26 in the House and 42-7 in the Senate in 2016. It allows for possession of a supply for 90 days, with the legal amount to be set at some point in the future.

26. **Pennsylvania**- In 2016, Senate Bill 3 legalized possession of a 30-day supply of marijuana with votes of 42-7 in the Senate and 149-46 in the House.

Legal Marijuana for Recreational Use

While the above states allow for marijuana to be used for medical purposes, very few allow it to be used recreationally. Without a prescription, you are can possess and consume marijuana in Washington, Colorado, Alaska, and Oregon. To grow marijuana for recreational use, you would still follow the same guidelines as anyone else in your state. If it is legal to grow as a recreational user, you will often need to fill out the right paperwork to become certified and then pay taxes on your crop. Some states even have programs in place where you can grow marijuana and sell it back to the state for profit.

Before you decide to grow in your state, find out what is legal. You should also consider your neighbor's and family's opinions before you decide how discreet you need your growing operation to be. The best way to grow marijuana is legally, so be sure to check out what qualifications you must meet in your state before you start growing your cannabis crop.

Step 2: Setting Up to Grow

Chapter 3: Deciding Whether to Grow Indoors or Outdoors

One thing that we can be grateful for during the marijuana prohibition is the new challenges that cannabis farmers were faced with. Since it was illegal to grow and sell marijuana, many marijuana farmers had to move their crop indoors. Now that restrictions on growing have been lifted in some areas, you have the option on relying on Mother Nature to do her job and grow outdoors or to make yourself a discreet, indoor setup. This chapter will help you decide what is best for you based on the level of discreetness that you need to achieve, the cost of setup and maintenance, and more.

Advantages of Growing Outdoors

In the days before marijuana prohibition, indoor growing setups were unheard of. This is likely because growing outside was convenient and easy, provided you could keep potential thieves and pests away. One of the major advantages of outdoor growing is the low maintenance. Instead of tending to your plants daily as you would need to with most indoor setups, you can tend to them 1-2 times weekly. The ventilation, light, and soil offered by the outdoors also mean that you have significantly cheaper start-up costs.

The other major benefit of growing outside is that it allows your buds to grow to their full potential when they are under the right conditions. This is likely because of the unlimited lighting and growing room, both to expand and grow upward. It is not uncommon for outdoor plants to get as high as 15 feet, with a big yield to go along with it.
In terms of flavor of the bud, it is up to your own personal preference. Some people swear by the quality of the bud grown inside, however, there are still many marijuana farmers and connoisseurs that swear by the flavor of outdoor buds. Marijuana outdoors has a wonderful flavor because of the unlimited sunlight, though this can be mimicked with expensive LEDs if you move your operation indoors.

Disadvantage of Growing Outdoors

While the yield that you get from growing outdoors is often larger than the one in outdoor setups, it is likely that you will only get one harvest per growing season each year, unless you live in a particularly warm environment. Additionally, while you only need to tend to your plant once or twice weekly, you will need to have a nearby source of water or risk lugging large buckets of water to your site. This is especially true if you have chosen a location that is off your own property.

The other major disadvantage of growing outdoors is the slew of outdoor factors that your plant may be exposed to.

This includes hungry bunnies, deer, and other pests, as well as humans that may come across your plants and try to take them. Additionally, you have to worry about them getting too much or too little water from drought or downpour, frost in the cold hours of the night, and possible bugs. If you take all the right precautions and choose a good location, however, you should be able to bypass some of these issues.

Advantages of Growing Indoors

As marijuana prohibition forced growers inside, they were forced to come up with more complex methods of planting. The good thing about this is that it allowed the development of higher quality marijuana strains, since you can control individual factors like the nutrient levels, light exposure, soil composition, and water amount for each plant. You can also use advanced methods to inter-breed different strains and tweak your method until you find the perfect levels for a specific strain.

Another major advantage of growing indoors is that you can grow the entire year. This allows you to grow strains in shorter strain and get a larger total yield from your crop. This, paired with the consistent quality of indoor buds, may even allow you to enroll yourself in a growing program where you can sell your homegrown marijuana back to the state for profit.

The final advantage of growing indoors is the high level of discreetness that can be achieved. Growing technology can even rid an area of marijuana aroma and keep your lights less visible to the naked eye.

Disadvantages of Growing Indoors

The major disadvantage of growing marijuana indoors, especially when you are just getting started, is the high start-up costs. You must provide the entire growing environment, including proper ventilation, the right lighting, water, soil, and nutrients. In addition to the higher start-up costs, you will need to consider the price of electricity for providing light to your plant every day and the slightly higher maintenance costs.

Additionally, while growing indoors is more discreet if you take the right precautions, there is no way to get out of trouble or claim the bud isn't yours when it is growing in your house. Of course, this won't be a problem if you are growing legally.

Ultimately, the decision to grow either indoors or outdoors is up to you. You should consider your budget, how discreet you must be, how many harvests you hope to have, and several other things before you make your decision. Since both methods have their advantages and disadvantages, only you can decide the method that is best for your personal operation.

The next three chapters will cover different types of growing. If you are growing outdoors, read Chapter 4. If you decide that indoor growing is your best bet, then you will want to read Chapter 5. Once you have the basics down, you may find Chapter 6 on growing hydroponically incredibly useful. This will teach you about growing in mediums other than regular soil and you can combine this with the information in Chapter 5 to create an incredible marijuana growing operation indoors.

Chapter 4: Setting Up for Growing Marijuana Outdoors

If you remember correctly, one of the biggest advantages of growing outdoors is that Mother Nature provides most of what you need for growing. This includes sunlight, nutrients, ventilation, and even water if the weather is just right. This makes it rather affordable to grow outdoors, however, there are still several things to keep in mind. This chapter will discuss choosing the right location, how to get quality soil outdoors, and how to test your water and nutrient quality.

Choosing the Right Location for Your Cannabis Crop

When you grow marijuana outdoors, it is exposed to many risks. To keep things such as pests, prying eyes, and the law away from your plants, it is important to choose the right location for growing your crop.

#1: Amount of Sunlight

The first thing that you should consider is sunlight. Even the plants requiring low levels of sunlight will need a minimum of 5-6 hours of direct sunlight every day. The best way to achieve this is to plant in an area that receives direct sunlight from the hours of 10 a.m. to 4 p.m. Any sunlight that is received in addition to this will just help your plant grow larger more quickly. You should also avoid planting near trees, hills, and buildings if you are worried about them blocking sun during some of the most critical hours.

#2: Level of Discreetness

Even if you are growing your marijuana legally, you may not want everyone to know about it. Some people still look down on marijuana use and others may try to take some of your crop for their own. You should remember that some marijuana plants can get quite tall when grown outside, even growing 15 feet or higher. Try to plant your cannabis in a fenced in area or surround it with trees or tall shrubs.

You also do not have to always plant in in-ground locations. If you do not have an area that is good to plant outdoors, consider placing a small plant in the window of your home or outside on a roof or balcony. If you are worried about being seen, you can easily place a few potted trees nearby to hide your plants from prying eyes.

#3: Access to Water

If you are worried about being caught with your marijuana crop for any reason, the best thing that you can do is plant away from your home. This could be a discreet location that nobody visits in your local woods or a nearby field that you have access to. Something to consider if you choose a remote location, however, is access to water. There are good odds that you will find yourself making a long trek with a lot of water if you plant in an area that is too remote and doesn't have any nearby lakes or rivers that you can borrow from.

#4: Exposure to the Elements

People are not the only thing that you must worry about when you plant your marijuana crop outside. Proximity to deer, rabbits, and other wildlife may find your crop tasty to munch on, while being planted at the bottom of a slightly downhill location can leave your plants susceptible to water damage or drowning. Consider the various elements that may exist in your area and then consider ways to protect your crop. If you are at risk from downhill water damage, then move to a higher location. Additionally, if deer and other munching animals are a problem, consider a growing cage or surrounding your plants with a fence to keep these kinds of pests away. For information on dealing with common pests, check out Chapter 13 on troubleshooting your grow.

#5: Temperature

If the temperature gets too hot or too cold a few days out of the month, your cannabis crop may not be as bountiful but it can still thrive. If you are worried about hot temperatures, be sure to plant away from bricks or concrete that will trap heat and radiate it into your plant. You should also avoid planting near surfaces like pools or ponds that will reflect the sun.

Ideally, cannabis should be kept in weather between 55 degrees and 86 degrees. If you are worried about your plants getting too cold at night, plant them near a brick wall or other surface that may have absorbed heat throughout the day. You should also consider the dampness or humidity in your area, because an area that is too wet without a good drainage system can cause mildew or mold to grow on your plants and can also cause disease.

#6: *Wind Exposure*

The right amount of wind provides good ventilation and can even cool your crop if you plant in a dry climate. It also increases water consumption, though, so be sure to give your plant plenty of water. If you are worried about too much wind, plant some windbreakers like shrubs or use a fence or decorative wall to protect your plants.

#7: *The Strain That You Are Growing*

The cannabis works like any other living organism- it must be able to adapt to the growing conditions of the area that it lives in to survive. Ideally, all the needs stemming from its original lineage will be met so that it can thrive and produce the best yield. You should heavily consider the climate of your specific area and what types of marijuana have been cultivated from climates similar to yours. You will find that some strains can grow in almost any environment, while those like Tropical Sativa can only be grown in the climate they are already adapted to.

Preparing the Soil in Your Garden

When you grow outside, Mother Nature provides soil that is often rich with nutrients for your cannabis to grow in. However, the nutrient levels and minerals in the soil are not always the perfect levels for growing marijuana. This section will teach you what you need to know to get the perfect soil for marijuana.

Balance of Soil Components

There are three different things that make up what we know as soil: sand, clay, and silt. When growing marijuana, having the perfect balance of these will give you proper drainage and ventilation for your crop to grow.

First, you need to understand the properties of each soil element. Then you can make changes to the soil so it is the right climate for cannabis to grow. These changes should be made about a month before you are ready to grow, especially if you are using materials that are going breakdown and absorb nutrients into the soil.

Sandy soils provide great ventilation and drainage, because the sand does not clump together. Unfortunately, everything runs through sand- including your nutrients. This becomes increasingly true in rainy environments or if you find yourself watering your plant frequently (which you should). If your soil is too sandy, dig out large holes in the area where you plant to have your garden and fill them with coco coir (made of the husk from a coconut), peat moss, and compost. These will add plenty of nutrients to your soil, as well as bind the soil together enough that there is good airflow and water drainage but nutrients are still absorbed.

Soils that are rich in clay are very heavy, which is one of the reasons that they do not hold oxygen to provide good ventilation and that they drain slowly. To improve soils that are heavy in clay, place decomposed organic matter like manure, worm castings, and compost and mix it in with the soil. This provides plenty of nutrients and will also break the soil up well enough that there is adequate drainage and ventilation.

Silty soil is by far the most ideal growing medium for marijuana crop. Silty soil can often be found in prehistoric lake bottoms and riverbeds. It is full of nutrients, holds moisture but also provides a good amount of drainage, and warms quickly to keep your plant's roots toasty on cold nights. This can be identified by its dark, rich color and crumbly texture.

Why pH is Important

The importance of the pH of your plant comes from the way that it absorbs nutrients. Each of the individual nutrients that a plant may need can only be absorbed at a certain level. When the pH is out of balance, your cannabis plant may not be absorbing one of the key nutrients that it needs. The result of this could be stunted growth, leaf discoloration, or any other symptoms that represent a nutrient deficiency.

For cannabis, the ideal pH for growing in soil is between 6.0 and 7.0. Marijuana grows best in slightly acidic soil. You can find this information out by sending out a sample of your garden soil for testing or by purchasing the equipment to test your pH yourself at home.

Consider Testing Your Soil

By far one of the easiest methods of figuring out the composition of your soil, as well as its pH balance and the nutrients that are in it is to send it away to be tested by a soil testing company. In addition to this useful information, you will find out if there are any contaminants like lead, pesticides, and other dangerous substances in your soil that may be leached into your marijuana plant. The report will usually be summarized with recommended nutrients to add to your soil. This gives you the option of either supplementing the individual nutrients that are missing or adding a fertilizer or nutrient solution that contains everything that your plants need.

If you find out that your soil is out of range on either the alkaline or acidic end before you plant, you can add things to the soil to raise or lower the acidity. You want to add a very small amount of the below materials to your soil at a time. You must adjust the pH slowly to get it in range, so start at least a week before you are ready to plant your cannabis. After you have added the small amount and mixed it through the soil, water it and wait at least a full 24 hours before checking it again.

If your soil needs to be more alkaline (if the pH is too low), you can add things like crushed marble, crushed oyster shells, hardwood ash, dolomite lime, or bone meal.

If your soil needs to be more acidic (if the pH is too high), you can add things like wood chips, peat moss, cottonseed meal, sawdust, or leaf mold.

Adding Physical Support for Your Plants

Your plant will benefit in a few different ways from a stake or growing cage. A metal or wooden stake (or even a section of lattice board) will provide your cannabis with support to grow upwards. Additionally, when you face harsh winds or heavy water droplets, they will not weigh your cannabis plant down. A cage works very much in the same way, however, it will give added protection by keeping out bunnies, deer, and other animals that may want to make your marijuana plants their next meal.

Additional Considerations for Growing in Outdoor Containers

You are not limited to planting your cannabis crop in the ground if you grow outdoors. Alternatively, you can plant in a bucket, pot, or other type of planting container. Then, these can either be planted directly in the ground with your plant or kept on a patio, in the woods, or anywhere else that you choose.

One of the major advantages of planting in an outdoor container is that you can transport your plant wherever you need to. This means that you can quickly move your grow operation if someone catches wind of your activities or you can bring your plants inside on nights where it gets too cold (and days where it gets too hot). The major disadvantage, however, is that you will not necessarily have as large of a yield as you typically expect from outdoor marijuana. This is because the size of your plant is limited to the size of the root system that can grow in your pot.

If you do choose to grow in an outdoor container, you can pick up special potting soil or amend the soil in your yard and put it in the pot. You can even collect soil from another outdoor area if you know that it is high quality (such as silty soil from your local riverbed). You will want to remember to choose a container with adequate drainage and plenty of airflow. For some containers, you will need to drill your own holes for aeration and be sure to choose a good soil. You can use perlite beads to improve aeration and drainage through your soil. You may also want to add rocks in a layer at the bottom of your planting container and put the soil on top of it.

Watering Outdoor Plants in Containers

You will likely need to water outdoor plants in containers more frequently than those planted in the ground. Depending on the heat in your area, you may need to water every day or more frequently. For potted plants, you want to thoroughly saturate the soil. Instead of watering on a regular schedule, pay close attention to the top one inch of soil. When it is completely dry, you will add more water to your plant and saturate the soil once again.

Once your soil has been prepared and you have all the things for your outdoor setup, you are ready to move on to the next step. If you know that you want to grow your plants outside, you can skip Chapters 5 and 6 as they apply directly to indoor setup.

Chapter 5: Setting Up for Growing Indoors

When you grow cannabis indoors, you must provide the entire environment for its success. This includes obvious things like "sunlight" and water, but also a growing medium, proper ventilation for your growing room and roots, and all the nutrients necessary for your marijuana to thrive. This chapter will teach you what you need to set up for growing indoors, from the different types of lighting to examples of systems that you can set up.

Start Small

Once you have made the decision to grow marijuana, it can be very easy to get wrapped up in all the excitement of testing your green thumb. However, even if you have the funds it can be a mistake to jump into a large growing operation right away. While you may be eager, mistakes that are often made by newbies can be quite costly and possibly cost you your entire marijuana crop. While reading this book will help you prevent that, it is still best to start with a few small plants (or even just one) to get a feel for what you cannabis needs before you jump into a large grow operation. Even though you are starting small, however, be sure to think big and choose a growing area that will accommodate a larger setup once you are ready.

Choosing Your Grow Area

The first problem that you must tackle upon deciding that you are going to grow marijuana indoors is where you are going to grow it. After all, even if growing marijuana is legal in your area, you will want to keep your operation a secret from most people, in case they blab to others or may want to steal your hard work. Some of the best places to grow in the house include a closet or cupboard, a spare room, or your basement. This section will go over the considerations that you must make when choosing the location for your grow space indoors.

#1: Discreetness

Even if growing cannabis is legal in your area, it is very likely that you want to maintain a high level of discreetness for your growing operation. For this reason, it is best to keep your grow area somewhere will people will not go unless they are invited. Once you have chosen a discreet location, be sure not to blab to everyone about it. Some people will just gossip about it when they run out of things to talk about, while others may find themselves brainstorming ways to get part of your crop. Only tell people that you trust the most and for the highest level of discreetness, tell nobody.

#2: Proximity to Electricity

Most people do not want to re-do the wiring in one room of their house for their growing set up. For this reason, you should consider the proximity to electricity before you choose your growing space. Your lighting system is going to need quite a bit of power, especially as your system starts to grow. Additionally, a closed indoor area often requires ventilation of some kind and this will use electricity as well.

#3: Ease of Cleaning

Cleanliness is a must when it comes to growing marijuana. Any unclean or damp surfaces can lead to mold and mildew growth and invite pests and fungus to live on your plants. If you do not catch it fast enough, you may have to dispose of your entire marijuana crop and start from nothing. To prevent this, make sure the area that you choose to grow in is easy to clean. Some of the most difficult areas to keep dry and clean are raw wood, drapes, and carpeting, so try to avoid rooms with these types of materials if you can.

#4: Keeping Light Brightness High

To mimic natural sunlight, your grow lights will need to be incredibly bright. Two things that will help you achieve this is having the right colors on the walls of your grow area and making sure that no light is escaping the grow area. You can either coat the insides of your grow area with Mylar or paint it with white paint. This will help to reflect light back onto your plants. You should also check for any holes, including cracks in doors that will let light escape your operation and decide what way to prevent light from escaping.

#5: Consider Humidity and Potential for Air Flow

Some climates and houses are naturally moister than others, which is a problem for cannabis plants. If you start with an area that is humid, you can expect to have problems in terms of humidity and may even need an expensive dehumidifier for your grow room. If it is an option, you should also choose a location with a window, smokestack, or other outlet to outdoors. If your cannabis operation grows, you may find the need to funnel the scent of your plants outdoors (through a carbon filter to mask the odor of course) or to use the outlet to let heat out.

Choosing the Right Container for Your Marijuana Plant

The right container is key to keeping your marijuana plant healthy and thriving indoors. There are several considerations that you must make, including the size of the pot, how the outside materials will conduct heat or cold, and how good the drainage and aeration is throughout the pot. If you are growing a single plant, then a simple pot with drainage will work well. You should also consider getting a pot made of a fabric outer, as this will allow incredible airflow for your plant.

Choosing Your Growing Medium

When you grow indoors, there are many different types of growing systems that you can use. For the most basic set-up, you are going to want to use soil. This can be basic, nutrient-rich soil from your local home and garden store because it will likely contain everything you need. Additionally, you will be able to adjust the pH using some of the methods from the previous chapter or by using a solution to raise or lower pH, which can be purchased at your local dispensary, online, or from select gardening stores.

Another option when it comes to growing indoors is hydroponics. These are soil-less techniques for growing marijuana. Some may make use of a soil-less growing medium like coco coir while others will use a drip system of water treated with nutrients to get your plants what you need. You will learn about hydroponic systems in detail in the next chapter.

Lighting

Obviously, you have the option of moving your marijuana plant around the house if you only have one to soak up sun throughout the day. For a little less work, it is very likely that you will want to try out one of the below types of lighting.

Fluorescent Grow Lights

CFL (Compact Fluorescent Lamp) bulbs are one of the lowest cost lighting options and a favorite of people growing on a smaller scale. They do not generate as much heat as bulbs used in larger grow operations and are typically more cost effective. If you are just starting out with a plant or two, then this is an excellent choice. You will even find a way to use this bulb to create an entire growing ecosystem with a few five-gallon buckets later in this chapter.

When choosing a fluorescent bulb, you want to choose one

with a high output. You will also find that proper reflective material is key to providing your plant with the amount of light that is needed to grow. They are not as efficient as some of the other options and generate around 25% less light for the energy that is used. However, fluorescent lighting does still have its benefits for smaller setups.

Fluorescent bulbs are also convenient, because all the parts necessary for you to grow your plants are included in the package, including the bulb itself, the reflector, and the ballast to regulate the flow of electricity and adapt your light to the environment.

A ballast is essential in many growing setups, because it will dim when necessary to save you electricity. You can also manually or digitally set some ballasts, which allows you to change the light at different times to mimic the natural growing season indoors.

HID Grow Lights

High intensity discharge lights are a very popular choice among growers because of their high output and great efficiency, as well as the value that comes when you bundle these two things together. They are more expensive than fluorescent options initially, but you will find your savings in efficiency and the total wattage used of electricity each month. Additionally, the high output of these lights allows them to be used for multi-plant growing setups.

When you grow marijuana, you will likely need two different types of lights. The first is MH, or metal halide. MHs give off lights that are a blueish white in color. They are used in the earlier vegetative stages of growth because they mimic the light of early Spring. The other HID light you will need is HPS, or high pressure sodium. This type of lighting is used in the later flowering stages, because the red-orange light that it gives off mimics the harvest time of autumn.

If you cannot afford both types of HID lighting, then you should start with HPS bulbs. These bulbs are the most efficient and you can still change the wattage when it is necessary to mimic seasonal changes.

Most MH and HPS bulbs do not come with a reflector/hood or ballast. The ballasts are either magnetic or digital. While you will find the magnetic more affordable, they are less efficient, get hotter, and will cause more wear and tear on your bulbs. If you do choose a better quality digital ballast, be sure to choose one that is high enough quality that it does not create an electromagnetic interference field.

LED Grow Lights

One of the more recent developments in indoor growing technology is light emitting diodes or LEDs. A high-quality LED setup has a few benefits, including more efficient use of energy, a longer life, and the creation of less heat. Some of the bigger, more efficient designs put off a full spectrum of light that allows for higher quality marijuana and bigger yields.

The downside of these fixtures is that they are often quite costly. You should also be very wary if you find a cheap LED grow light, as there are many manufacturers that offer less than quality products. These will not be able to do nearly what you want to with your marijuana grow. Always be sure to read reviews online and if any seem like they are overly positive, do a check with the Better Business Bureau to be sure the site hasn't been reported for poor service.

Other Lighting Consideration

Something else to consider as you set up your lights is their initial height and their final height. As you make your system, remember that your plants are going to grow. The best light systems will allow you to adjust them per the height of your plant by raising them up. You may even be able to achieve this with a few clamps in the right places if you are tight on funds.

Ventilation

If you remember grade school science class, then you already know that carbon dioxide is one of the critical components of the photosynthesis process. This means that your plants will need fresh air to let them thrive. The best way to do this is to provide a steady stream of air through your grow room. Regardless of your setup, you can put an exhaust fan pointing outward to blow through your grow area. This is best placed toward the top, since hot air rises. A second exhaust outlet should be positioned pointing inward toward the bottom of the grow area, across from the first. This will create a steady flow of cool air in and hot air out. You will find this is also useful for regulating the temperature for your plants.

Temperature

For cannabis plants to engage in the natural growing process like they would outdoors, you must regulate the temperature in your grow room. If you know the specific strain that you are planting, then you have the option of looking up the best temperature for that strain. In general, marijuana grows best at temperatures between 70 and 85 degrees Fahrenheit during the "daytime" lights and between 58 and 70 degrees at "night", when lights are off.

Adjusting the Temperature for Your Specific Strain

The best temperature for a marijuana plant is that found in its natural climate. Indica strains typically prefer a cooler temperature, while Sativa strands often come from warm and even tropical climates. The best thing to do is buy a specific seed type and do your research on its preferences, however, you can shoot for an average if you do not know what you are working with.

Often, a grow room will regulate its own temperature based on the amount of heat that your lights give off and the size and position of your exhaust fans. Before you set everything up, turn on the lights in your room and see what temperature it rises to after a few hours. Adjust your exhaust fans accordingly, until you have created the perfect environment for your cannabis.

Regulation

One of the most critical pieces of the growing process

overlooked by new cannabis farmers are the tools necessary for regulation of your plant's environment. It is important to remember that you are going to be out living life while you are waiting for your marijuana plants to grow. This means you will not always be around to adjust the temperature in your grow room or turn the lights on and off to mimic the natural grow cycle.

A very useful tool in this case is a timer. A timer can be used for the lights to give them the ideal amount of "daylight" before it is time to sleep. When used with a digital ballast, they will also be able to adjust the wattage based on the time of the day.

You can also set up the exhaust with a timer, to help cool down the room at nightfall. Alternatively, you can set up a thermostat to work with your exhaust fan. The exhaust fan will turn on whenever the room starts to get too hot. It costs a little more, but it is well worth it and will be more energy efficient in the long run.

DIY System: Space Saving Marijuana Bucket

If you are trying to create your first growing system, this bucket is a great place to start. As you put it together, you learn about all the important parts of a growing setup, including lighting, proper ventilation, drainage, and more.

Necessary Materials

- 4 5-gallon buckets (white, 1 with lid)

- 4 CFL lights (23 watts) and included adapter

- Power strip

- 12V 2A power supply

- 2 PC fans

- Mylar (or another reflective, non-conductive material)

- 8 ¼ inch wood screws

- Heat-resistant glue or other bonding material

- Zip ties

- Black duct tape

You should also have a drill and/or screwdriver, and either a Dremel tool or a knife that is sharp enough to cut through the thick plastic of a 5-gallon bucket safely. A marker will also help with more precise cutting.

Instructions

The first thing that you are going to do is prepare the bucket where your plants will live. Use the drill or Dremel tool to put drainage holes into the bucket. Then, position one of the fans on the upper part of the bucket and trace it, being sure that it is positioned so it will blow on your growing cannabis plants. Then, cut out the area where the fan will be placed. This will provide the fresh airflow and oxygen that your plants need.

Next, put the fan into place. If it is not tight enough, you can use some heat-resistant glue to seal any gaps. Take the zip ties and use them to secure the power strip to the outside of your bucket.

To prepare the drip pan, you will start by measuring 3 ½ inches from the bottom side of the bucket. Use the market to make a line and space out the 8 wood screws, spacing them as easily as you can. Measure an additional 3 ½ inches above this line and cut the top off the bucket.

You will also have a light top, which will hold the bulbs for your plant. Consider where the light adapter that you are using will fit most appropriately on the lid and cut this area out. Then, assemble your lights so they are positioned in the middle of the lid. You are also going to trace an area for the exhaust fan in the lid, so it will blow heat out from the lighting and help suck the fresh air from the lower exhaust fan from the bucket. Place and seal this the way you did the first PC fan.

Finally, take the two extra buckets that you have. Measure 1 inch below the lowermost ridge on your bucket. You will set aside the tops of these two buckets to add to the top of your space bucket as your plant grows. These will let you raise up the lighting so your plant does not get too hot. Additionally, it allows you to grow taller plants than you typically can with this system.

Assembling the Bucket

To assemble this setup, simply put the main bucket into the drip pan. Connect the exhaust fans to the power supply and hook your lights into the power strip. Add your rocks, potting soil, and plants and then put the light on top. Don't forget to add the additional bucket tops for added height once your plants begin to grow.

Advanced Technique: Creating an Artificial Environment

This is an incredibly advanced growing technique, so we will not go into details here. It is also quite expensive and hard to maintain, so it is not a good choice for someone just starting to test his or her green thumb for cannabis. It is, however, an interesting concept and it is something that you can consider putting together once you hone your marijuana growing skills.

An artificial environment will be completely sealed and there will be no exposure to the elements. The climate is typically regulated in these types of grow areas using many timers and various measuring tools, a dehumidifier, an air conditioner, and a system to supplement CO2.

Chapter 6: Growing Marijuana Hydroponically

Another frequently used method when growing marijuana indoors is hydroponics. Hydroponically grown marijuana describes a growing process done without soil. Instead, a soil-less growing medium is used. This chapter will review the considerations that you must make when growing with a hydroponic setup. You can combine this information with what you learned in the previous chapter about indoor growing to produce higher quality buds.

The Major Advantage of Growing Hydroponically

Like all other methods of growing marijuana, a hydroponic setup has advantages and disadvantages. The major advantage of hydroponic growing is the incredible amount of control that you have over your growing system. Soil itself is an ecosystem, meaning that you must deal with the pH and nutrient levels of the soil, as well as changing bacteria levels that may affect your plants. You must deal with the levels for your plants, as well as the ever-changing soil and that can be difficult. When you grow hydroponically, it is incredibly easy to control the temperature, pH, and nutrient levels of your entire growing environment. This allows you to produce a consistently good harvest of marijuana.

So, What Do You Need to Set Up Your Own Indoor Hydroponics System?

Though the techniques used vary, there are some basic pieces of equipment that you will need for your hydroponics system. These include:

- Grow Lights- Unless you have an incredible amount of sunlight in your grow area (which is usually unlikely for indoor growing), you will need grow lights for your operation. Keep the considerations from the last chapter in mind as you choose your lights.

- Growing Chamber- Your growing chamber describes whatever part of your system where your roots will grow. For some systems, this will be an entire tray. For others, this will be netted pots or other growing containers. As you consider the growing chamber that you will use, you should consider how much light your container will attract or deflect, as well as whether it provides both good aeration and good drainage. Something else that you must consider is the size of your containers. Your marijuana plant will not be able to grow larger than the root system, so the amount of room that your roots have is key.

- Reservoir- The reservoir describes the part of your system that holds your water/nutrient solution. This will either run through a drip system, pump the solution into your growing containers, or work with another hydroponics technique. You will learn more about the various hydroponics systems a little later in the chapter. Remember to keep your reservoir very clean and to change out your nutrient solution whenever it is needed.

- Delivery System- The delivery system is going to vary based on the technique that you choose. For the most part, it will be made up of PVC tubing or piping and connectors. The only thing that will be different is the size of the pipe and where you need to connect it for your particular hydroponic growing system.

- Submersible Pump- You can usually find these in home improvement stores or in hydroponic supply shops. In a home improvement store, they may be sold as pond or fountain pumps. You will need to adjust the pump in relation to the size of your growing operation. Another necessary part of a submersible pump is a filter. If your choice does not have one, you can easily make one yourself by cutting a small piece of screen or furnace filter. Make sure that you clean your pump regularly, because a blockage could damage your entire growing operation.

- Simple Timer- While your marijuana plant is growing, you are going to live your life. This means that you will not be sitting around the house all day to switch your plants lights and nutrient solution on or off. Additionally, cannabis requires very precise timers to produce a quality product. This is where timers come in handy, because they can be connected to your lighting system, your nutrient system, and your submersible water pump. You can choose analogue or digital, though a digital can wipe your settings if it loses power and cause your growing operation to dysfunction.

- Air Pump (Optional)- Some setups use an air pump, which supplies a great deal of oxygen to the water. This is set up by attaching a line to air stones. The air pump will push air through the line and then create oxygenated bubbles that rise through the nutrient solution. These are generally only used for water culture systems.

Choosing Your Growing Medium

Hydroponically means without soil. So, what do you grow marijuana in, if not soil? This section will teach you about the many growing mediums for hydroponic cannabis.

Soil-Less Growing Mediums

For a growing medium to be considered soil-less, it will not have a pH or other factors that affect the growing environment of your marijuana plant. This will allow a greater control over your environment. Here are some of the most common soil-less growing mediums for growing cannabis:

- **Coco coir**- Coco coir can be found in any DIY store, as it is a very popular growing medium, both alone and mixed in with soil or perlite. Coco coir is made up of the brown, fibrous husk of the coconut. For growing cannabis, a good way to use coco coir is to mix it coco coir with a ratio of 75% coco coir and 25% perlite. This can also be used with soil, to loosen the soil if it is compacted too much.

- **Rockwool**- Rockwool can be purchased from most home improvement stores. It is commonly used for hydroponic tomatoes but it can work just as well with cannabis. Rockwool is a manmade material that is made by melting down basaltic rock and adding it with thin fibers. This mixture is quickly cooled to form slabs, cubes, and even granulated materials. It provides excellent retention of water and good airflow, so it is optimal for your marijuana plant. It is commonly used in hydroponics setups, since it is used as an alternative to soil during the germination process.

- **Poprocks**- These are harder to find than other options and your best bet is to search for them online and see if there are any near you. These are smooth, round balls that are made up of shale that has been formed into pellets with a super heating process. These expanded clay balls are very easy to clean, which makes them reusable. When used in a hydroponics setup, poprocks provide perfect aeration and flow of water because they do not absorb water at all. They also come in different sizes. Poprocks only need to be rinsed well before you use them.

- **Lava rocks**- You can find lava rocks in most landscaping areas of home improvement stores. They are big, red rocks that are porous. However, they do not absorb water and provide airflow, which makes them a good growing medium. If you are expecting large plants that may shift lighter growing mediums, these are an excellent choice. You can also use them as anchors for stakes, drip lines, air stones, and more. To get lava rocks ready for your marijuana plants, you need to soak them for 3-5 days. You also need to rinse them off before use.

- **No Growing Medium**- Another alternative is to use aeroponics or a nutrient film technique, both of which will be discussed in the next section.

Techniques for Growing Marijuana Hydroponically

Another way to grow hydroponic plants is without use of a growing medium. Instead, your set up will involve adding the nutrients directly to your water (as you would with even a soil-less growing medium) and then using a drip system or misting the roots of your plants to help them get the nutrition that they need to thrive. This section will go over the basics for different types of hydroponic techniques.

Nutrient-Film Technique

When you use a system that does not use any growing medium like the nutrient-film technique (NFT), you will find that it is nearly impossible to end up with pests. You can also avoid mold and mildew growth by keeping your growing area and water reservoir clean. An NFT system makes use of a continuous flow of nutrient-rich water. This is fed to your plants and then drips back into a reservoir, which will then be used again. The other major benefit of this is the amount of water saved, because all unused water is cycled back into the reservoir to be used again.

Aeroponics

An aeroponics system makes use of net pots for growing your plants. These are positioned over a misting system and the roots of the plant are sprayed with the nutrient-rich water at set intervals. This reduces waste and saves you electricity by being set on an interval. Additionally, there is very little chance of your roots developing root rot and most types of fungi.

Wick System

The wick system is not a good idea for large plants or plants that have a high demand for water. This system works with a growing medium. Your plants are potted in the growing medium and then you run a wick from the materials down into a nutrient-rich water solution. The wick will transfer this into the growing medium so that it can be absorbed by your plants.

The key to success with a wick system is aerating your water. You will want a submersible pump or another aeration system to be sure you are getting enough oxygen into your water. This will also help to prevent mold growth.

Drip Irrigation

The goal of drip irrigation is to provide just enough water and nutrients for your plants to thrive, minimalizing waste. It works by feeding nutrient-rich water solution to a drip system that is set on a timer. Your plants will be fed at set intervals, getting just enough water and nutrients for its health. A drip irrigation system can be used either with soil or a soil-less growing medium.

This is a very low maintenance way of growing. If the temperature and humidity of your grow room is ideal and you have a large nutrient reservoir, you could even go days without checking in on your system. As an added benefit, this minimizes your need to interact with the ecosystem and reduces the chance of your presence disrupting the growing environment.

Deep Water Culture, Bubbleponics, and Recirculating Deep Water Culture

Like many other hydroponics water systems, these options allow the roots of your cannabis plants to come into direct contact with the air that contains the oxygen they love so much. This is accomplished using a reservoir that is filled with a pump to create air bubbles, plenty of nutrients, and water.

For this type of setup, you suspend the net pots from the lid of a 5-gallon bucket (or another container). You will germinate your plants in rockwool or another material before transferring them to the net pot. The roots hang directly into the nutrient solution. An air stone and air pump are used to create bubbles in the water, providing plenty of oxygen in addition to the other things your cannabis plant needs to grow.

Bubbleponics and recirculating deep-water culture systems are more advanced forms of deep-water culture. Bubbleponics is a large-scale deep-water culture system with a pump that feeds nutrients, air, and water through the top of your reservoir. Recirculating deep-water culture systems has a separate reservoir that attaches to several buckets and plants.

Ebb and Flow Systems

Ebb and flow systems are a more complex system that require a close eye. The reason is because it contains many working parts, all of which must be functioning to prevent slow growth or even death of your marijuana crop. Clay pebbles or poprocks are a good choice for this type of system, but they must be small enough to allow even distribution of the nutrients and water.

This particular setup involves a plant tray that has buckets suspended over it. When the timer goes off, your nutrient solution will flood the plant tray for a set amount of time, allowing your plants to soak up nutrients. Then, the solution is drained into a reservoir where it can be used again.

Adjusting the pH of Your Water Supply

Most soil-less growing mediums are neutral, meaning they do not affect the pH of your plants growing environment. The important levels of pH for this type of growing set up, therefore, must come from the water supply. Like when growing in soil, maintaining the right pH range is essential to getting the nutrients your plants needs and preventing vitamin deficiencies. This is because nutrients are only able to be absorbed within a certain pH range.

The ideal range of pH for cannabis when it is grown

hydroponically is 5.5 to 6.5, which is slightly more acidic than cannabis grown in soil. You will want to let your pH balance set on both sides of your spectrum, closer to 5.5 on some days and closer to 6.5 on others. This is because some of the nutrients only absorb at the more acidic side of the spectrum and others absorb closer to a neutral pH level.

There are a few different methods for adjusting pH of your water.

If you are doing a traditional hydroponics setup and need to raise the pH, you will want to use potassium silicate. If you are using a bioponics or hydroorganics setup, then you will want to add lime or sodium bicarbonate to make your water more alkaline.

To lower your hydroponic pH or make it more acidic, you will use a substance depending on the stage your cannabis plant is in. For a vegetative stage, you should use nitric acid. For the flower stage, you should use phosphoric acid.

The Germination Period

When you use a soil or soil-like medium, you can plant your seed and wait for it to grow (or wait for it to sprout a taproot first). For most hydroponics set-ups, however, you must germinate the seed before planting. Rockwool works well for germination. You can even use a rockwool tray, if you are trying to germinate several plants at once. You will learn more about germinating your seeds or clones later in the book.

Now that you understand the basics of indoor growing and

hydroponic, we will discuss your next option that you must consider- whether to use a seed or a clone to start your plant. From there, you will learn about nurturing either a seed or a clone through its early stages into a healthy young plant and from there to a fully budded marijuana.

Step 3: Choosing and Nurturing Your Seed or Clone

Chapter 7: Starting from a Seed vs. Starting from a Clone

When you have your setup ready and you have collected most of your growing materials, you are ready to decide whether you would like to start from a seed or start from a clone. This chapter will teach you about the advantages and disadvantages of each choice. Then, you can read on to chapter 8 on seeds or chapter 9 on clones depending on your choice.

Advantages of Growing from a Seed

The advantages of growing a seed vary depending on where you source your seed. If you choose a high-quality seed bank, then you have the option of choosing guaranteed feminine seeds, which means you won't have to weed the males out once they start to bud. Another option when you buy from a seed bank is auto-flowering seeds, which will begin to grow within 2-4 weeks if you expose them to a lot of light. To determine how high-quality a seed bank is, you can check the reviews on their website. If their reviews seem overwhelmingly positive, check with the Better Business Bureau to get the real story on the company.

Another benefit of growing from a seed is that you get a clean start regarding pests or disease, whereas clones may carry a predisposition to complications from the mother plant. Additionally, if you know the strain, then you can find out information like what the bud will look, taste, and smell like, how long it will take to reach maturity, the quality of the bud, how much a typical yield is, and specifications about growing conditions. Finally, after your first few times growing you can mate a male and female plant to produce seeds that are crossbred of whatever strains you choose.

Disadvantages of Growing from a Seed

There are also a few disadvantages to keep in mind if you are using a seed. First, while you can get auto-flowering or feminated seeds from a seed bank, seeds are not guaranteed to germinate. If you choose convenient bagseed, then you have this risk as well as not being able to know whether they are male or female, how well they have been stored, or the quality of the bud.

Another drawback of growing from a seed is that they take longer to grow, though you can shorten this with auto-flowering varieties. Seeds can also get quite expensive, especially if you choose specialty seeds or want to purchase famous strains. If you plan ahead, however, you can get male and female seeds in famous brands to breed your own seeds when you are ready.

The final thing you must consider is the discreetness of the shipping process. There is a potential of packages from seed banks being stopped at the customs border but you can buy from a company within your country or choose one with a very discreet shipping process. Adding additional items to your order to make the seeds less noticeable can also help. You can also consider purchasing from a dispensary.

Advantages of Growing from a Clone

When you grow from a clone, you cut a section off a mother plant. Then, you will tend to it until it grows a root system and eventually flowers into bud. One of the main reasons that people choose clones is because there is a guarantee of quality. If you know the lineage and health history of the mother plant, then you know the quality. There is also no guesswork concerning gender, so you are guaranteed a female plant.

Another benefit of growing from a clone as opposed to a seed is that you will be able to harvest sooner, shortening your total growing and curing time by weeks. If you can procure rooted clones, you will be able to shorten this process even more. These are also easier to stabilize and more likely to grow.

Disadvantages of Growing from a Clone

While the fact that your clone is going to inherit its genes from its mother is an advantage, it also means that the clone can inherit disease from the mother or a predisposition to certain kinds of pests. Additionally, the genes will change with time, including the possibility of the strain to lose strength. You can cross breed or interbreed a new clone into the system if this happens.

Something else to consider is sourcing your clone. This is difficult because mailing a clone can cause it to go into shock. Some clones even die in the traumatic shipping process. You also can get a clipping off someone you can trust or buy from the dispensary, but this is not always an option.

Additionally, clones are very sensitive after being planted even when they are in the best of conditions. Even the slightest mistake on your part can cause the clone to go into shock, which will stunt its growth.

*Note: If you are a new grower (as it is assumed you are since you are reading this book), it is a good idea to start from a seed first. Clones are very picky and can be hard to raise to a rooted phase, especially if you do not know what you are doing. It is advisable that you get some practice with seeds before moving on to growing from a clone. Additionally, if you find a strain that you like, you can raise it to be a mother plant so you do not have to worry about sourcing your clone.

Ultimately, the decision to grow from a seed or a clone is your own personal choice. You should consider how much you are willing to invest, your skill level, how quickly you would like to grow your plant, and whether you are growing outdoors or indoors before making your decision. Since each method has its advantages and disadvantages, only you can determine what is best for your growing set-up.

Chapter 8: Choosing and Nurturing Your Seed

When you are ready to grow your seed, you will still need to make a few considerations. This includes figuring out where to source your seeds from, how to select the best quality seeds for growing, and how to store your seed until you are ready to plant it. This chapter will teach you all you need to know to choose the best seeds for the best possible chance at growing a thriving cannabis plant.

Where to Find Seeds

You have three common options for finding seeds.

First, you can purchase from a qualified online seed bank. The major advantage of this option is that if you work with a trustworthy company, you can be guaranteed the quality of your seeds. Be sure to use an authorized seed bank however, instead of a black-market dealer who may be lying about where the seeds came from.

You also have the option of automatic flowering and feminized varieties. Another place that you may be able to find seeds is a dispensary. For states where growing is legalized but dispensaries are not common, however, this can be a difficult feat.

Your final option for sourcing your seeds is to choose bagseed found in the sacks that you purchase. While finding seeds in hydroponically grown marijuana is incredibly rare, you will have better luck finding them in lower quality weed. You may also find someone willing to pollinate one of their females to produce seeds for future growing. The downside of bagseed is that you cannot choose the gender, nor can you always determine the quality or lineage of the seed.

How to Tell if Your Seeds are Quality

The key to a great cannabis harvest is starting with a quality seed. There are a few characteristics that you should consider, including:

The color of the seed. A good marijuana seed will be a shade of brown or gray, or a combination of the two. Additionally, the surface of the seed will be glossy. You should avoid those that are light green or white, because these are often too young and will not germinate.

The pattern of the seed. Some marijuana seeds will have a uniform color, though most will have tan, brown, or black marks or lines on the outside of the seed. If your seed does have a pattern, it should be distinct. A blurry or unclear pattern is often indicative of a seed that has not matured all the way.

The hardness of the seed. Once marijuana seeds reach the point where they are ready to grow, they will not crack when you put slight pressure on them. Place a seed between your forefinger and thumb and apply a light pressure. If it does not crack, then the seed is hard enough. Be sure not to use too much pressure, however, because even the best seeds will crack if enough pressure is applied to them.

The size of the seed. As cannabis seeds mature to the stage where they can support the life of a future cannabis plant, they will plump up. For this reason, small seeds typically do not have the plant matter necessary to germinate a healthy plant. Choose large, plump seeds for the best chance at germinating and growing a thriving marijuana plant.

The shape of the seed. Marijuana seeds typically have a teardrop-like shape. They also are oblong, instead of round when they are more likely to germinate.

Extra Tip for Testing Bagseed

Sometimes, you may be questionable about an entire batch of marijuana seeds. If you keep all your seeds from a select source in one spot, you will be able to test the quality by breaking open a few of the good seeds in the bag. Randomly select a few good looking seeds and crack them open. Taste them and smell them to determine the likely quality of the rest of the seeds in the bag. Here is what you are looking for:

- A seed with a musty smell or taste and oily feeling is close to going bad. They may still germinate, but the growing process might be slower than you expect.

- A seed with a blackened appearance is already going bad. This blackness is caused by the fermentation that will likely prevent the seeds from germinating.

- A dusty and pale appearance on the inside indicates an old seed. This may survive the germination process, but will probably produce slow-growing low-yield plants.

*Note: If you would like to check the odds of your seed germinating before you plant them, stick all your seeds in a bowl of distilled water. Those with a large mass will sink and these are the ones that you want. You must do this just before you are ready to grow your plants, since marijuana seeds must be kept completely until they are planted to remain viable.

Proper Storage

You can choose to purchase seeds before you are ready to use them. If you keep them in a dark, cool place ten you may find that they produce quality bud for a couple years. Your refrigerator will even work. After this time, however, they can start to age and then they will grow more slowly, even in the most ideal of conditions. You should also remember that proper storage is key to keeping a seed fresh for years.

How to Germinate Your Cannabis Seed into a Plant

The key to getting your cannabis seed to germinate is the

proper balance of water, air, and heat. There are a few different methods that can be used for germinating marijuana seeds to get them ready to plant. This chapter will teach you a basic method that will work for most plants and then additional steps that should be used to give your seeds the best odds of germination.

Steps for a Basic Germination

All you need to know to germinate most seeds is the quality and amount of water necessary, a good amount of aeration, and a warm enough climate for them to grow. This section will break these things down. You may notice that light is not included on this list- this is because light is not required in the earliest stages of germination. Cannabis seeds in nature germinate even when they are covered in dark soil.

Heat- Your source of heat will be your own personal preference, but you can use a heated chamber, a hot light, or just regulate the temperature of your growing area. Something to be cautious of is regulating your heat source. A temperature between 75 and 80 degrees is ideal. You will find that lower temperatures encourage fungal growth and slow down the speed of seed germination, while temperature that are too hot will slow down the germination process as well.

Water- Water is an essential ingredient to start the germination process because it triggers hormonal changes within the embryo of the plant. Unless you use the below method of germination, you will want to choose rockwool or a top-quality soil to start growing in. If you do choose soil, be sure that it is pH balanced around between 6.0 and 6.5 and has good drainage. You will want to maintain constant moisture by watering frequently. This water will be absorbed through the shell of the seed and reach the inside, where the dormant hormones will be activated. Eventually, these hormones will cause a taproot to grow. Bottled water is the ideal choice for watering germinated seeds, because it is free of chlorine in city water and dissolved solids in well water.

Oxygen- The final ingredient in the equation to give your seed life is plenty of air. The roots like oxygen and the leaves take in carbon dioxide. In addition to these parts of air being necessary for growth, a good airflow will help prevent too much humidity. Humidity can pose a problem because it causes stem and root rot, fungi growth, and other potential problems that can stunt your cannabis plant's growth or even kill it entirely.

Rockwool cubes and other well-draining, aerated mediums are ideal for the germination process. If you choose a material that you will not be using in your actual growing setup, you can easily transplant the seeds using the right technique once they have sprouted. If you are worried about transplanting, consider taking the additional steps below to help ensure an easy germination process.

Additional Steps that May Help Old and Other Troublesome Seeds Germinate

If you are unsure of the age of your seed or how easy it will be to spur growth, there are steps that you can take to make it more likely that your seed will germinate.

1. Start by scuffing the seed slightly. Take and emery board, sandpaper, or sand and scuff a few tiny scratches in the outer shell of the cannabis seed. Be

very careful that you do not penetrate so deeply that you damage the inner embryo of the seed. This will make it easier for water to come through the outer hull to nourish the embryo inside.

2. Next, pour a bottle of water into a bowl and allow it to warm to room temperature. Soak your seeds for as little as two hours, but not more than 24 hours. This will soften the outer shell and make it more likely that the embryo inside will burst through.

3. Then, layer a paper towel on a dinner plate or in a container. Place the seed on top of the paper towel and then take a second paper towel and layer it over the seed. Take bottled water and pour it on the paper towels, being sure to thoroughly saturate the paper towels. To prevent your seeds from drowning, tip the plate to about a 45-degree angle and allow it to drain off.

4. You will want to keep your seed in a warm place (between 75 and 80 degrees) for a few days, until you can see a small green shoot protruding from the shell. You can regulate the temperature of a grow area or use lighting. If you do use a heat source, be sure to wet the paper towel as needed to keep the seed moist.

5. Once the tap root (this is the small green shoot) appears, you should place your seed in another growing medium immediately. A pH balanced soil or rockwool that has been soaked for the appropriate amount of time is the best choice, because they are well aerated and drain properly. You will learn about the specifics of this process in the next section.

Planting Your Cannabis Seed and Caring for It

Once you have completed either the first or second set of instructions, you will be ready to place your germinated seed in a growing medium to sprout. The ideal medium is either rockwool or well-aerated and well-hydrated soil. This should be kept at a pH between 6.0 and 6.5, to ensure that your plant has the best chance of absorbing the nutrients necessary for it to thrive. You will also balance the pH of your water out to this range.

If you are using rockwool, you will begin by soaking the cubes in a solution of lukewarm water that has been adjusted to a pH of 5.5. This will adjust the pH of the rockwool. Allow it to soak for at least one hour and remove it from the water. Place it on a rack so it can properly drain and then flush it with fresh water that has also been adjusted to a 5.5 pH level. Next, use a screwdriver or pencil to create a small hole in your growing medium that penetrates to about half of an inch deep. Take a pair of tweezers and gently pick up your sprouted seedling. Place it into the hole that you made with the taproot pointed downward. Use loose rockwool to cover the seedling and wait for it to grow. Be very cautious as you cover the seed, however, because a seedling will not be able to break through solid rockwool.

If you are using soil, start by filling a small pot with a potting soil with a light and airy consistency that has been adjusted to a pH between 6.0 and 6.5. Press it down gently, not packing it solid but compacting it slightly. Use the end of your finger to make a small hole in the center of your potting container, about half of an inch deep. Drench the soil with water that has been adjusted to a pH of about 6.3, allowing it to absorb the water without making it waterlogged or soggy. Then, use a pair of tweezers to pick up your small sprout and place it with the taproot pointing downward in the hole that you made. Use loose soil to gently cover the seed.

*Note: It is very important that you do not use a pot too large for your small seedling. While replanting later may seem like a hassle, having a small pot is essential for proper drainage. Using a pot that is too large makes it difficult to fit your pots on a heating pad and can also encourage the growth of mold, mildew, and other fungi.

Once you have planted your seedling in soil or rockwool, the only thing that you need to do is keep it wet. After 2-5 days, the seeds should have sprouted up through the growing medium. In most cases, they will shed their shells and reveal the oval-shaped leaves of their embryo. In some cases, the leaves of the embryo are not yet strong enough to remove their shell. Be patient, but if it is unable to do this itself you may be able to use a small pair of tweezers to help them along. If you do choose this method, you will find that it is incredibly easy to kill the seedling.

Once the embryo has emerged, position your plants under your growing setup, being sure that the lights are close enough to provide sunlight but far enough away that the heat does not damage your cannabis plants. Set your lighting timer so that your lights have 18 hours of daylight and 6 hours of nighttime.

The timing with which you will start adding nutrient solution to your plant will depend on your growing medium. If you started with a seed grown in soil, you should wait until your plant is at least 1 week old before adding any nutrient solution. Then, add a 20% strength nutrient solution directly to the water supply before you water your plants. If you planted your seed in rockwool, which has no nutrients of its own, you can start adding a diluted nutrient solution of 20% (or less, to be safer) as soon as it is potted. Since seedlings are still sensitive, however, many people opt to wait at least a week before starting to feed their plant.

For your seedlings to have the best chance to grow, keep them at a temperature between 75 and 80 degrees, as you did during the germination process. They will require a much lower humidity, however, within the range of 20-40%. To keep them from contracting fungi or disease that could kill them, do not allow the humidity to rise over 55%.

Once you have made critical decisions about your seed and know how to test for quality, you can move on to germinating it with your setup. If you want to learn about growing clones, move on to the next chapter. If you are certain you are going to use seeds (at least at first!) then feel free to skip ahead to the next section on the growing process.

Chapter 9: Choosing and Nurturing Your Clone

The clone process starts with a cutting made from the end of a branch that is growing out a new set of leaves. This cutting, or clone, is then planted. With the right conditions, it will start to grow roots and eventually flower into a budded marijuana plant. Clones are incredibly sensitive after they have been cut so it is important that you have a good understanding of how to care for one before you take your first cutting. Here, you will learn just that.

Taking a Cutting

In some cases, you may source your clone from another person or a dispensary. In this case, you will not need to do the cutting yourself. In an ideal situation, you will be sourcing your clone from your own marijuana plant. This is the best choice because you know exactly where the cutting came from, the quality of the mother plant, and whether the mother had any pests or disease that could be passed on to the clone.

Necessary Materials

Here are the various items that you will need to clip your clone and start the rooting process:

- A mother plant

- Scissors

- A scalpel or clean razor blade

- Ceramic dish or other cutting surface

- 1 cup lukewarm water in a glass

- Rooting powder or gel

- Plastic spray bottle (with mist setting)

- Propagation chamber (heated)

- Growing medium (rockwool cubes or trays work great)

Instructions

You are going to want to start by adjusting your water pH so that you give your clone the best possible start. Adjust it until it is within a range of 6.0 and 6.5. Then, add the water to your growing medium. If you are using rockwool cubes, you will need to soak them at least 20 minutes beforehand so they are saturated thoroughly.

As you are waiting, you are going to make your cut. Take the scissors and use them to make cuttings from the mother plant at the end of branches that have a minimum of 3-4 leaf nodes growing from them. Ideally, the mother should be a few weeks into the growing process but not yet flowered.

Once you have your cutting (or cuttings) take the scalpel or blade and use it to trim all the leaf nodes except those at the very top from the cutting. Make your incisions as close to the stem as you can without causing damage. You should be sure to make this cut at a 45-degree angle. Then, scrape away the outermost layers of the plant (bark) away from the bottom to reveal the inner stem.

Next, prepare the powdered or gelled rooting solution and dip the bottom of the clone into it, being sure that the lowermost one centimeter on the clone is thoroughly saturated. Next, take the rooting blocks from the water and squeeze gently. You will want them to remain wet, but you do not want them so soaked that they are dripping. Insert the tip of the stem into the block, being sure that the clone root is at least 3-4 centimeters below the surface. Stick this in the heated propagator (the heat is optional, but you will still need a propagator for your clones to grow).

Read on to the next section to learn about maintaining the health of your clones. Your cuttings should have roots that are visibly coming from the root blocks in 2-3 weeks, at which time they will be ready for transplantation.

*Note: Even under the best circumstances, cloning can fail. This is especially true if you do not know the exact type of your plant and do not understand its natural growing climate. For this reason, it may be a good idea to take several clippings from your mother plant at once in case some are unsuccessful. This lessens the likelihood of wasting a few weeks if your clone is unable to grow roots.

Tending to Your Clone to Raise it to a Healthy Sprout

There are several different parts to clone maintenance if you want it to live long enough to grow a root system and eventually develop into a fully budded cannabis plants. This section will teach you how to raise your clone to a sprout.

Temperature, Humidity, and Lighting

As an average, clones will root best in temperatures between 68 and 78 degrees. This degree range is not excessively hot, nor is it excessively cold. For clones to develop a root system, they must remain plump and moist. This is the reason that you should keep them within a humidity range of 90-100% for at least the first few days. You can cut back the humidity later to prevent problems with root rot and other fungus, but do not allow the humidity to drop below 60-70%.

When you first cut your clones, you can either put them in 16-hour per day light with the mother plant to prevent them growing too fast or move them immediately to a system of 12 hours on and 12 hours off.

The Key to Preventing Mold, Root Rot, and Fungus: Ventilation

Another essential part to developing a healthy sprout from your clone is ventilation. If you have already been growing, then it is likely your current exhaust system is strong enough to remove moisture and add fresh air to your marijuana plant's breathing area. This will prevent stem and root rot, gray mold and other disease, and fungal growth.

In addition to proper ventilation, you can prevent problems like mold, root rot, and fungus by doing two other things. First, you should ensure that no part of your root system is ever submerged in water. This will prevent it from draining properly and can create excess moisture. Second, you should be sure that your growing medium is incredibly well aerated and that it drains well. This is one of the reasons that rockwool is preferred as growing medium for clones for many professional growers.

Caring for and Nurturing Your Mother Plant

If you keep trying your luck at cloning until you get it right and you find a marijuana strain that you love, you can keep this indefinitely as a mother plant. The technique that you will use to keep your mother plant alive will depend on your particular setup; however, you will need a separate area and lighting system for your mother plant. You will keep it alive with a growing medium (or hydroponics system), nutrients, and water as you would any other plant in your cannabis crop.

The key to maintaining a mother plant for use of future

cloning is preventing it from flowering. A cannabis plant can be tricked into growing indefinitely if it never reaches the flowering stage of its life cycle. This can be accomplished by making the plant live and grow under a light system that is on for 16 hours and off for 8 hours. The longer "day" that your plant is living will keep it in the vegetative stage indefinitely.

As you try your green thumb at clones, remember that they are incredibly picky about their environment before rooted and even the best growers sometimes have difficulties with their clones. For this reason, always be sure to take several cuttings. Additionally, once you learn more about the lineage of your mother plant, do the research to provide an environment more suited to the strain for an increased chance of success.

Step 4: The Growing Process

Chapter 10: Nurturing Your Cannabis Crop from Sprout to Maturely Budded Plant- Growing in Soil

If you followed the tips for either your seed or clone and have raised them to have a root system and they are now at least a few inches tall, then there are good odds you are on the right track. This chapter will go over the considerations for what you should do after your seed or clone has become a young cannabis plant and help you nurture it to a full-grown bud, whether you are growing indoors or outdoors.

Planting Your Sprout

If you used a small pot for starting the growth of your marijuana plant or you started your plant as a clone or seed indoors and want to move it to outdoors, you will need to re-plant your marijuana sprout.

If you are growing outdoors, be sure that the soil of your ground has good drainage and aeration and that it is pH balanced before you try to transplant your sprout. Start by digging a hole that is a little bigger than the size of your pot. If you want to allow unlimited root growth and encourage a larger plant and bigger yield, you will want to very carefully remove your plant (and the soil surrounding it) from the pot. Place this in the hole and cover with loose soil.

If you are growing indoors and you want to move your sprout to a larger container to maximize growth, you should apply the same technique as above. However, instead of digging a hole, start by removing your potted plant carefully from the pot and placing it in the middle of the new growing container. Surround it with nutrient-rich soil to give it the best chance at growing.

Choosing the Best Soil for Replanting

When you grow in soil, the method of adding nutrient solution to your water used in hydroponics is not the most cost-effective or efficient method of giving your plants nutrition. Instead, you will want to choose the right soil to make sure that your marijuana plants get the nutrition they need right away. The best way to get fertilized soil is to start with a pre-fertilized super soil. Ideally, this will be an organic, homemade blend that you have made yourself.

The reason that homemade blends are preferred over store bought brands of nutrient-rich super soil is because the blends of nutrients found in store bought brands will not necessarily suit a cannabis plant. A skilled grower who knows the balance of nutrients needed by plants (you will get there one day with practice!) may be able to purchase pre-made fertilizer because they understand what cannabis plants need to thrive. To make a homemade, organic super soil for your garden, mix bat guano and a small amount of worm castings in your soil

Providing Your Plant with Nutrition

Once your plant is in the ground, you will need to replenish the nutrition of the soil from time to time. To do this, you have a few different options, including organic fertilizers, nutrient solution, and store bought fertilizer.

Organic Options

When you have an outdoor setup, fertilization is often the chosen method of providing your plants with nutrient. Soaking your water with nutrients is just not a viable option when you have such a large area that you are working with because the nutrients will spread out to the close areas of ground and much of it will go to waste or be soaked up by other plants. The ideal type of fertilizer, therefore, is a homemade blend that supplements exactly what your soil needs to nurture a marijuana plant.

Typically, everything that you need to support a healthy, thriving cannabis plant can be picked up at your local home and garden store. The key is knowing which ingredients do what and then mixing them together in the right amounts to create the perfect mix for your plant. Think of this as a science. While cannabis plants are not overly picky, learning the right blend for your strain will give you a healthy plant and incredible harvest. Here are some of the most popular organic additives for your cannabis garden and what they contain:

Blood Meal

Blood meal is not a vegan-friendly garden additive, but it boosts the nitrogen content of your soil incredibly easily. Blood meal is made of the blood from animal packing plants, especially cows. It is dried and then turned into a powder. In addition to adding nitrogen to the soil, it will raise the acidity so you should use at a time when you need a slightly lower pH balance.

If you use blood meal, be sure to closely follow the instructions printed on the bag that you bought, as increasing the nitrogen level too much can prevent your plants from developing buds and even has the potential to burn your plants and kill them. In some areas, blood meal also can be used to deter deer, moles, and squirrels because they find the smell of blood meal unappealing, making them less likely to choose your marijuana garden for a snack. However, it can also attract carnivorous animals like possum, dogs, and raccoons.

Additionally, if you find that you have an ethical issue with where blood meal is sourced, there are also the options of feather meal or alfalfa meal. You can purchase blood meal and possibly alternatives from large home improvement stores, though you will get a more affordable price at feed stores and local nurseries.

Bat Guano

Bat guano is another word for bat droppings, which have been collected from the bottom of a cave where a group of bats live. It is well known by expert growers of cannabis and many other gardeners who choose a more natural route for fertilizing their plants. Bat guano is incredibly rich in phosphorus, though it is a slow release as it breaks down. While you can use it periodically as a fertilizer, you will ideally add a good amount to your soil before you start growing.

In addition to being high in phosphorus, bat guano does other things for your plant. It is also high in calcium, which helps stabilize the pH of soil. When mixed into soil, it improves soil structure, water retention and nutrients, and oxygenation. Finally, it has a reputation for leaving a natural, sweet taste to the crops that are sometimes referred to as a 'touch of mango'.

Kelp Meal

Kelp meal is derived from the kelp that you find in the ocean. It is dried and then ground into a powder before hitting the shelves as a fertilizer. The major benefit of kelp meal to your marijuana plant is potassium, though its benefits do not stop there. The ocean is full of trace vitamins, minerals, and nutrients, which are leached into the seaweed as it soaks in it throughout its life. When it is dried and powdered, it retains these benefits.

As a standalone fertilizer, kelp meal should be added in a dosage of ¼ cup per plant for full-strength fertilizer. If you are using it combined with other ingredients for your soil, you will need to balance out the separate ingredients to find the optimal soil fertilizer.

Worm Castings

Worm castings can be thought of as a miracle fertilizer for

your soil. Worm castings are incredibly rich in vitamins and minerals and it has several effects on the soil where your cannabis plants will grow. Here is a breakdown of what it can do:

1. **It removes heavy metals from organic waste**. When you have heavy metals in your soil or fertilizers, it can stop your plant from absorbing some of the key nutrients that it needs to thrive. Worm castings balance the level of heavy metals, so that the nutrients found in the worm castings are released periodically through the growth cycle of your plant.

2. **It fixes the carbon-nitrogen balance of organic matter**. When you grow organically, it is not uncommon for the balance of carbon and nitrogen to be 20 to 1, or even higher. Adding worm castings to your organic mix balances this. It reduces the carbon levels, which is essential because a carbon level that is too high can lead to a soil that is more acidic than you would like. It also raises the nitrogen levels, so it becomes more available for your marijuana plants.

3. **It increases water retention in the soil**. When worm castings are added to soil, they form mineral clusters known as aggregates. These aggregates prevent the soil from eroding away from the water and compact it more. They also increase the soil's ability to retain water.

4. **It purifies the soil by removing harmful toxins, fungi, and bacteria**. When you add worm castings to your soil, it removes these things and makes it less likely that your plants will develop

certain plant disease. This is because of a compound known as humus that is found in the castings.

5. **It contains humic acid that stimulates growth of your marijuana plants**. When humic acid is introduced to the soil of an area, even in small amounts, it boosts plant growth. The reason that humic acid can be introduced in such small amounts is because it is found in an ionically distributed state. This makes it very easy for the roots of your plant to absorb.

6. **It prevents extreme pH levels**. Balancing the pH of your soil is a fine art, whether you are indoors or outdoors with your plant. When you add worm castings, a protective barrier is made around the roots of your plant that protects it from pH levels that are either too high or too low.

Fish Meal

Fish meal is not necessarily the preferred fertilizer for some marijuana growers, but it does work. This organic choice is high in the nutrients nitrogen, phosphorus, and potassium, with a ratio of 10-2-2. It is also high in macronutrients and micronutrients, contains plenty of vitamins including B-complex vitamins, and contains all the necessary amino acids that your plant needs to thrive. This works very slowly, so it is best to put it into the soil about a month before you plant your cannabis. It will take 30-60 days to break down so you may want to apply over the life cycle of your plant. Additionally, it helps build the soil if it is too crumbly to hold water well.

Bone Meal

Bone meal is an organic fertilizing option made from the bones of animals, typically those from meat packing plants that would throw them away anyway. These bones are steamed to clean them and remove any undesirable residue. Then, they are crushed into a fine powder. Bone meal is ideal for the same reason as blood meal - it contains plenty of phosphorus. You will find that it is essential for the development of healthy roots and flowers later in the growth cycle. Bone meal also contains a good amount of phosphorus.

Bone meal slowly releases with time, but you must use it in small quantities. One half of a teaspoon is a sufficient amount for 2 square feet of soil or one plant. Mix this into the top 1-3 inches of soil before you plant your plants.

Nutrient Solution

The good news is that if you buy a nutrient solution especially for marijuana, you will not have to mess around with mixing your own solution. This is an incredibly fine art that should be only attempted by someone who has a good idea of what their plant needs, especially if you start with a medium like soil that already contains its own nutrients. You must be especially careful with phosphorus, since there is a chance that it can burn your cannabis plant's roots in high concentrations.

Choosing Store Bought-Fertilizer

If you look at the contents in a pre-made fertilizer, you will see plenty of nutrients, vitamins, and minerals that your plant needs to thrive. Unfortunately, unless you buy fertilizer that is manufactured especially for marijuana plants, you must be careful about balancing these with the nutrients contained in your soil. This is the reason that store-bought fertilizer is often chosen by more experienced growers that know exactly what their plants need to thrive.

If you do choose a store-bought fertilizer, be sure to closely follow its instructions to avoid harming your plant. When it comes to gardening, even the slightest miscalculation can damage your harvest. You should also be wary of potential pesticides in products, because they will be leached into your marijuana plant and can affect the taste and the aroma.

What Your Marijuana Plant Needs to Thrive

If you are going to attempt mixing your own organic fertilizer or nutrient solution or attempt to buy store-bought fertilizer, it will be important to know which vitamins, nutrients, and minerals that your plant needs.

The key to marijuana growth is the correct level of phosphorus, potassium, and nitrogen. All three of these will help to produce strong roots for cannabis plants that will be able to suck up plenty of nutrition, large leaves to collect light and make food for your plants, and lush flowers that will produce high-quality, high-quantity yields.

When your plant is in the first 2-3 weeks, most potting soils will have enough nutrients for what it needs. Once the leafing and the vegetative growth cycle begin, you will want to add enough potassium, phosphorus, and nitrogen to provide your soil with a 20% concentration of each. This is only true when you are growing outdoors, however. If you are growing in a container, you may want to cut this back to only ½ or even ¼ of the recommended dosage for 20-20-20 solution of these three minerals. If you notice any leaves drooping on your indoor plant, there is a high likelihood that you added too much solution and your plant went into shock. In most cases, you should provide your plant with nutrition about twice a week. Some outdoor growers, however, administer these nutrients daily since they often spread into the surrounding soil.

Once you have reached the point where your plant is ready to flower (this will depend on your lighting cycle and if your plant is ready to produce bud), you will need to increase some nutrients to your plant and decrease others. You will also need a larger variety of nutrients than before. You should feed your plant phosphorus, potassium, and nitrogen in a 30-10-10 ratio. The secondary foods for your plant include magnesium, sulfur, and calcium. These may be found naturally in your soil or potting soil, but you may need to supplement them. The easiest way to find out what you need is to have your soil test. Finally, you will need trace minerals including manganese, zinc, copper, iron, molybdenum, and boron. These are only needed in small amounts, but you will want to balance the pH of your soil as well to ensure your plant is absorbing them.

Removing the Males from the Grow Area

Cannabis plants can be either male or female. The male plants are used for hemp, while the female plants flower and produce the marijuana that can be smoked or turned into a non-smokeable form. If you buy genetically engineered female seeds or opt for a clone, you will not have to worry about removing the male plants from the growing area.

If you want to produce the highest quality marijuana that you can grow, you do not want males in your growing area. This is because when female plants are exposed to males, they can be pollinated. This causes seeds to form within the buds of the plant, lowering the quality by medical and recreational standards.

When to Remove Male Cannabis Plants

In the vegetative stage of growth, marijuana plants will typically have a very similar appearance to others. This means that it is nearly impossible to tell whether you are dealing with a male or female plant at this stage. For some plants, they will reach a pre-flowering phase at about six weeks of age. If you look in the area where the stem connects to the leaf nodes, you will see little "pre-flowers" forming. The sign of long, wispy white hairs instead of the development of pollen sacs (this is what the male produces) is a good sign of a female plant.

For other marijuana plants, you must wait until the flowering stage to find out whether your plant is male or female. It can be exhausting to watch all of your hard work turn out male plants, which is the reason that many growers choose to clone their cannabis or purchase feminized seeds. Once your plant reaches the flowering stage, you will notice the appearance of either long pistils that will turn into marijuana buds (on females) or small ball-like plant parts that will turn into pollen sacs (on males). This can be tricky to tell in the earlier stages, but you are guaranteed to be able to tell by the time your plant has been in the 12-12 lighting phase for at least 1-3 weeks.

Something Else to Watch Out For: Hermaphrodites

Something else that you must be cautious of is plants that appear as if they could be female, but are actually hermaphrodites. These types of plants have some female characteristics, but they develop secondary sex characteristics that allow them to pollinate the females. If keeping your plants seed-free and high quality is important to you, these must be removed from the growing area as well.

There are two things that you should watch for to tell if your plant might be a hermaphrodite. As the buds start to grow, you will notice the stamen typically found in the male pollen sac growing on the outer part of the bud. These must be removed almost immediately, because a stamen does not even need to produce pollen to pollinate your female plant. Another sign that you must watch for is the appearance of long, yellow, banana-shaped growths. These are frequently referred to as "bananas" and failure to remove these can also result in seeds in your female plant.

How to Remove Unwanted Plants

Once you have identified the plants that need to be removed to stop them from contaminating your harvest, you will need to remove them in a specific way so that there is no chance of re-growing. If you have planted your marijuana in separate containers, then you will not have to worry about this because you can easily dispose of the unwanted plant. If you are growing them all in a large system or growing outside, however, you will need to manually remove the entire male cannabis plant. Dig down deep into the soil around the undesirable plant, being careful not to cut into the root systems of neighbor plants. Then, remove the bulb of the plant and as much of the root system as you can. If a few weeks pass and you see new growth, remove them immediately since the plant that has regrown will be the same sex as its parent plant- male.

Watering Your Marijuana Plant

The cannabis plant requires plenty of water, which makes sense when you consider that marijuana plants contain 80% water. It is also the lifeblood of the plants, necessary for nearly all the life processes that the plant will go through, including transpiration and photosynthesis, keeping the leaves stiff and healthy, and nutrient uptake. This makes giving your plant the right amount of water to help it thrive, without providing so much that your plant's roots are drowning in it.

Choosing the Right Water

When you water your plant, the water you use will depend on your area. While purified water is a good choice, you must also be careful because the reverse osmosis process that is typically used to purify water also takes out the naturally occurring nutrients. If you find that you must use purified water, be sure to test the nutrient level of your soil and fertilize or add nutrient solution as necessary to keep your plant healthy and thriving.

If you live within city limits, you will likely find that you can use your tap water. Before use, however, be sure to test it for contaminants from metals and other sources. You should also check the pH, though this can be balanced if you need. The easiest way to balance the pH of your water is using a solution sold in many home and garden sections to either raise or lower your ph. Another issue with city water is chlorine, however, chlorine will dissolve when exposed to air. Collect the water for your marijuana plant at least 24 hours beforehand and allow it sit in an open container to dissolve all of the chlorine.

If you live outside of city limits and have well water in your home, then it is very unlikely that you will be able to use your water source. This is because well water often has dissolved solids in it that can harm your plant. If you find yourself needing to use purified water, that is okay. Just remember to supplement the nutrients that you need to and balance the pH before you use it.

Frequency of Watering

The key to watering marijuana is finding the perfect balance between under watering and over watering. Skilled growers know that you must have at least a small dry period so that your marijuana buds can reach maximum potency and have an ideal growth. If you allow your plant to get so dry that the leaves wilt, however, you need to replenish your plants water immediately.

The frequency that you will need to water your plants will depend on whether they are grown inside or outside, the size and age of your plant, and the container that it has been planted in.

When your plant is a seedling, it will need plenty of water to encourage growth but this must be provided in incredibly small amounts to stop the seedling from drowning. Consider taking a small spray bottle and misting the soil around your plant, being cautions of the stems and leaves. This will prevent hot light from being attracted to the water droplets on the plant and possibly prevent burning.

The amount of water necessary for your cannabis plant during the vegetative stage will depend on the efficiency of your setup and the size of your plant. Additionally, plants in smaller containers will need watered more frequently than those in large containers, because you cannot give them as much water in one dose without causing the soil to be waterlogged and risky your plant being drowned. When you are growing in containers, you should check the first centimeter of your soil. If it is dry, then you will want to add water. This could be once a day or more often in some conditions. Once they enter the flowering stage, you will find that your plants are absorbing more water to grow the buds. Continue to add water as often as necessary and check frequently to make sure that your plants are getting what they need.

If you are growing in the ground outdoors, you will sometimes be able to take advantage of groundwater or rainwater and water your plant less. You should still be sure to give your plant plenty of water. You can do this by feeling the top one inch or so of the soil. When it is completely dry, you will give your plant more water. In-ground, outdoor plants will usually need watered a few times a week, while those in containers will need watered more frequently. Do not be worried if you are doing this often, a large cannabis plant is capable of drinking as much as ten gallons of water every day!

Providing Lighting for Your Plant

If you are growing outdoors, then you do not have to worry about much concerning lighting. If you chose a bright, sunny location when you planted your cannabis crop, the wonders of Mother Nature will take care of all the lighting specifications for you. It will grow your cannabis into a healthy plant during the vegetative stage and eventually, as the days grow shorter, it will be coaxed into a flowered marijuana plant.

If you are growing indoors, then having a timer is essential to preventing unnecessary stress on your plant so that the light comes on and shuts off at the same time each day. The amount of lighting necessary for your plant will be determined by what stage it is in. In the earliest days of your plant, after the leaves have started to show, you will want to give your plant about 18 hours of light per day. Once it begins to flower (or you are ready to coax it into flowering), you will want to provide it with 12 hours of light per day.

Another thing to consider is whether you purchased auto-flowering seeds. If so, the amount of light can be kept at 24 hours per day and they will still grow into an abundant harvest.

Now that you have reached this chapter, you should know everything that you need to take a seedling planted in soil to a point where its ready for harvest. Best of luck if you are going to use this method- and be sure to check out Chapter 12 on troubleshooting your grow BEFORE you get started so you can pinpoint common mistakes and how to avoid them.

Chapter 11: Nurturing Your Cannabis Crop from Germinated Sprout to Maturely Budded Plant- Growing Hydroponically

This chapter will provide you the basics for growing hydroponically, though you should note that you will need to adjust your methods slightly depending on your growing material and the setup of your situation. If you have been following the instructions in this book, you will have either a seedling that has been planted in rockwool material or a clone that is planted in a hydroponic growing medium. Either plant should be a few inches tall and have a strong root system when you are ready to start nurturing it to grow into a plant.

Removing the Males from the Growing Area

Once your plant starts to flower, you will want to remove the males from the growing area (if there are any). You can tell if a plant is a male because it will develop a pollen sac at the area where the marijuana branches off, instead of a long pistil. You also must be wary of stamens or banana-shaped growths on buds, because these indicate a hermaphrodite plant that can cause your female plant to seed. These do not need to be open to pollinate, so you will want remove them immediately. This type of plant can even cause itself to seed.

Providing Your Plant with Nutrients

The genius behind most hydroponic setups is that they take soil out of the equation. Unfortunately, most hydroponic systems do not trap nutrients well because they run down through the growing medium, often into a reservoir that helps to recycle the nutrient/water solution. Other setups may mist the roots of the plant with water or use a system where roots hang in the water filled with nutrient solution and bubbles provide your marijuana plant with air.

Regardless of the set-up you choose, the nutrients of your plant should be provided through its water. In the earliest stages, you will want to use a N-P-K (nitrogen, phosphorus, potassium) solution made especially for hydroponics. This nutrient solution can be measured and then added to your water. This can be continued through the vegetative stage, following the dosage instructions on the bottle to prevent harming your cannabis crop. Once your plant moves into the flowering stage, you will find that you need a high amount of phosphorus and lower amounts of potassium and nitrogen in a 30-10-10 ratio. In addition to the NPK nutrients, your plant will also require fair levels of sulfur, calcium, and magnesium. Trace amounts of zinc, boron, iron, manganese, molybdenum, and copper are also needed for the best buds.

You will want to stop providing your plant with nutrient solution about 1-2 weeks before you are ready to harvest. Since there is no soil to absorb the extra nutrients in the water, your plant will likely absorb them. Many people find that this leaves them with a chemically aftertaste when they smoke them. As an alternative, use plain water that has been pH balanced to provide your plant with nourishment. You should also note that it is normal to see older leaves turning yellow or even falling off. This is a result of the plant relocating the nitrogen that has been stored in the leaves to the buds of your marijuana plant.

Watering Your Marijuana Plant

When you grow hydroponically, there is a very high likelihood that you will have a timer set up so you do not have to think too much about watering your marijuana plants. The key, therefore, is being able to calculate how much water your plant needs and when. Then, you will pump it full of the recommended amount of nutrient solution for its growth cycle and leave it up to itself.

The best way to adjust your watering cycle is to monitor it closely. Your water will likely be set on a timer for a hydroponics system. Start with once or twice a day and watch between cycles. To prevent mold and mildew growth and plant disease, you will want to allow your growing medium to dry 30-50% before watering it again. The amount of time will vary based on the strength of your exhaust system, the amount of heat that your lights give off, the temperature of your growing area, and the stage of growth that your plant is in. Remember that you should set your timer to water your plants more frequently during the flowering stage because then need more water to grow bountiful buds.

Providing Lighting for Your Plant

In the earliest stages of germination, providing your plant with light is optional and only necessary if you intend it to be used for heat. Once the cannabis plant is starting to sprout, put it under a light for at least 18 hours per day. Follow this regimen through the entire vegetative growth stage.

You will know that your plant is ready to start flowering when it has reached half of the height that you intend it to. This can change depending on the strain, so do your research if you can. The average half-height for a hydroponically grown marijuana plant is anywhere from 6-18 inches, especially in a limited space like a cupboard or closet.

Once your marijuana plant has reached the right height, you will want to switch it to a cycle of 12 hours with light and 12 hours without. This will stimulate the days of fall and help to coax your plant to flower.

If you have reached this point, then I want to wish you luck with your hydroponic practice. Remember that growing marijuana hydroponically is a fine art and you should not be discouraged if you do not have a bountiful harvest right away. Once you do reach the level of skill where you can grow hydroponic bud to harvest, head over to the next step to learn how to harvest, dry, and cure your marijuana for smoking. If you had any problems, check out the next chapter on troubleshooting your grow.

Chapter 12: Troubleshooting Your Grow

Even if you do all the right research and be incredibly cautious as you start growing marijuana, you can still make miniscule mistakes. Additionally, things out of your control may happen that will affect your crop. This chapter will teach you all about troubleshooting your grow and how to deal with nutrient deficiencies, pests, fungi, molds, disease, and more.

Identifying the Problem

The key to troubleshooting problems that you may be having is identifying the symptoms. Here are some of the most common problems that you can have with your plant and how to identify them:

Watering Problems

You can either underwater or overwater your marijuana plants (unless you have the perfect balance, of course). There is a very subtle difference between these conditions. If you overwater your plant, the entire plant will wilt and you will notice the leaves drooping downward. If you underwater your plant, the entire plant will look like it is wilting and the leaves will look lifeless and limp, instead of just drooping downward. They will be much less lustrous than if you overwater. You can easily fix this by monitoring and regulating your water cycle.

Nutrient Deficiencies

Often, discoloration of your marijuana leaves (among other things), are the cause of nutrient deficiencies. Here is what to look for:

- **Magnesium Deficiency-** This will appear in the older leaves, found on the lowermost part of your cannabis plant. You will notice significant yellowing between the veins.

- **Zinc Deficiency-** This will cause the tops of your leaves to yellow.

- **Sulfur Deficiency-** This will cause the lowermost leaves of your plant to turn yellow. The damage will start at the base of the leaf and slowly spread to the tip before moving up the plant.

- **Iron Deficiency-** This deficiency causes the inner leaves and topmost leaves on your plant to turn white or yellow.

- **Boron Deficiency**- This deficiency causes brown spots, accompanied by new growth on your cannabis plant that is excessively thick, twisted, or otherwise abnormal.

- **Manganese Deficiency**- This deficiency causes mottled brown spots on leaves. You will also notice yellow between the veins on your leaves.

- **Potassium Deficiency**- This will cause the outer edges of your leaves to turn brown or yellow. You will also notice yellowing a little further in.

- **Calcium Deficiency**- This causes brown spots and stems that are hollow or weak.

- **Phosphorus Deficiency**- The colors associated with phosphorus deficiency can vary, but you will notice strange coloring of your marijuana plant leaves. Then, dark splotches will appear and the leaves will eventually fall off the plant.

- **Copper Deficiency**- You will watch the upper leaves to see this deficiency. They will become very dark in color and the edges and tips will turn yellow.

- **Molybdenum Deficiency**- This appears as either pink or red coloring on the leaves of your cannabis plant.

The solution to this one is easy. Simply identify the problem and then balance it with the right nutrient supplementation.

Nutrient Abundance

Too much of anything is bad, including nutrients. The most common problems are general nutrient burn and nitrogen toxicity. Nutrient burn will appear as brown tips on your plants and the leaves will eventually burn all the way down and fall off without remedial action. Nitrogen toxicity will appear as dark green leaves, with the tips turning downward into a claw shape. If you catch this early enough, you can just reduce the amount of nitrogen (or nutrients) you are feeding your plant. If you still have problems with it, try flushing your growing medium with fresh, pH-balanced water.

Pests, Bugs, Mold, Mildew, and Viruses

If you have any of these symptoms, mold, mildew, or virus may be to blame:

- **Mealy Bugs-** These are not particularly small, so if you notice a hairy bug crawling on your buds and/or leaves, it may be mealy bugs.

- **Leaf Miners-** Leaf miners live inside of your leaves, so they will be hard to see. You will, however, notice light green or white trail-like patterns on your leaves and possibly holes from the critters munching.

- **White powdering on leaves-** If you have a white substance that looks somewhat like flour, white powdery mildew may be the cause.

- **Barnacle Insects**- These stick under leaves and plants and will be noticeable as they sap your plant's nutrients.

- **Leaf Hoppers**- These come in a variety of colors, but they are noticeable by the speckled pattern that they leave behind on the leaves of plants.

- **Spider Mites**- If your plant has spider mites, you will notice small white speckles. If you have a decent sized infestation, you will notice spider-like webbing on the underside of your leaves.

- **Snails/Slugs**- These will come out only at night and eat your plants, leaving holes in the leaves and slime trails behind.

- **Aphids**- Aphids will live under your leaves, sapping the nutrients of your plant. They have different life cycles, so it's hard to say what they will look like.

- **Russet Mites**- These mites are nearly impossible to see, so you will notice twisted, blistered, and glossy leaves after their visit. Your buds may also turn brown and the plant will grow poorly.

- **Leaf Septoria**- This is a type of fungus that will cause yellow and brown spots on the lower leaves of your plant.

- **Fungus Gnats**- These love a moist environment, so if you have these tiny, dark flies and a sick plant, you may want to dry your growing medium better.

- **Whiteflies**- You may see these tiny, moth-like creatures if you look under your leaves.

- **Tobacco Mosaic Virus**- Though this is more likely to affect tobacco plants, this disease can affect cannabis as well. It causes bright yellow, splotchy spots on leaves.

- **Thrips**- Silver spots, spittle, or 'snail' trails are indicative of thrips. If you can find the thrips themselves, they will look like tiny worms.

In any of these cases, a targeted approach is best. Do your research and find a method of treatment. If you can, aim for an organic treatment that will not affect the quality of your marijuana buds. You should also be sure to clean any equipment or growing medium that has been used while your plant was infected/infested.

Other Problems

The major other problems that may affect your plant include root rot or other root problems and pH fluctuations. In any of these cases, the lowermost leaves will appear as brown or tan spotting. Start by checking and balancing the pH levels of your plant. Then, if you can see the roots of your plant, inspect them closely. Since all types of fungi, parasites, and bacteria can affect and kill your roots (and your plant), it can appear differently. In most cases, however, the roots will be slimy. To prevent root rot, you can try topping off your reservoir instead of changing it when your plant is young. You can also cool your grow room a little, increase aeration, or a root-friendly bacteria supplement. Damaged roots and leaves will often not heal, so sometimes it is best to start over!

Bud rot is another problem that you may experience, which can be devastating to a new grower. There is no coming back from bud rot, so the most you can do is isolate the bad buds and decrease humidity to decrease the likelihood of your other buds getting infected. Your buds will start to look sickly and become discolored and if you open the bud up, you will find that it is moldy or dead.

Tips to Stop Potential Problems Before They Start

#1: Test, Test, Test

One of the biggest mistakes that new growers make is overlooking the importance of regular testing of pH, nutrient levels, temperature, and humidity. These things all have the potential to cause problems for your cannabis plants if they are not addressed immediately. Before you start growing, invest in a thermostat for your grow room (preferably one that regulates the exhaust system), a pH testing kit, and a humidity test strip. You may also find it useful to send out your water and your soil for testing (if you are using your own from home) so that you can remedy any imbalances or contaminants before you get started.

#2: Carefully Regulate Your Temperature

Failure to regulate temperatures can be a huge problem for marijuana plants. Not only will it disallow the abundant harvest they can produce, it causes unnecessary stress on the plant. Too high of a temperature also means that you may need to water your plant more. The problem with this is that your plant will be taking in extra nutrients with the water, which will burn the tips of the leaves if you do not regulate the problem immediately. If your light being too close is the problem, you will notice wilting and either browning or bleaching of your plant.

#3: Proper Ventilation is Key to Success

You should never underestimate the power of a good ventilation system. Your system should be effective enough that it removes moisture from the air and quickly replaces it with fresh air, to keep your plants both cool and dry. You do not want so much ventilation, however, that your plants dry out very quickly and need more water. The reason that proper ventilation is so important is because it prevents a moist environment that promotes bug infestation, mold and mildew growth, and other problems.

Step 5: Drying and Curing Your Marijuana Buds

Chapter 13: Harvesting, Drying, and Curing Your Marijuana Buds

Congratulations! If you have reached this chapter, then there are good odds that you have used the information in this book to successfully grow some marijuana! The good news is that your buds are done. The bad news, however, is that you cannot smoke them just yet. First, you must dry and cure your marijuana buds to make them the perfect moistness and maximum potency for smoking.

When to Grow (and Harvest) Your Marijuana

Growing Outdoors

For most outdoor growers, they can harvest once per year by following the natural growing cycle of a plant. They plant their cannabis in early spring, once the frost has stopped at night. Then, the plants thrive and grow all the way until the early days of fall.

As you choose when to grow your cannabis, consider the

legality of growing in your area. Law enforcement knows that a May-August growth cycle is common for marijuana plants, so they will be on the lookout for it around this time.

Growing Indoors

One of the biggest benefits of growing indoors is that you can harvest year round. Therefore, the determination of when to grow and harvest your marijuana will depend on your own personal preferences and how much you are trying to grow yearly.

Signs That Your Plants are Ready to Harvest

You will know that your cannabis buds are ready to harvest by paying attention to the pistils and the trichomes. The pistils are the hairs on the outside of the bud. You should aim to have at least 50-80% of these hairs an amber/brown color before you harvest. You will also want your trichomes to change color. These will be clear as your plant is growing. When your plant is ready to harvest, either half will be milky-colored and half will be amber or all the trichomes will be milky colored.

You should also be aware that you can change the way that your bud affects you by changing the harvest time. When you harvest earlier, you have more of a Sativa effect on the body that allows for a thoughtful, in-your-head high. If you are seeking for a body high like you would get from an Indica plant, then you will want to wait to harvest until a little later. You can experiment with harvesting times on the same strain of bud until you find what works best for you- then stick to it!

Harvesting and Drying Your Marijuana Buds

When you are ready to harvest your buds, you will need a sharp pair of scissors. You can either cut the plant above the roots or cut off the buds individually, leaving a few inches of stem below them so you can hang them. Once you have cut all the buds off, trim the leaves. You can save these in a separate area if you plan on using butter, hash, or another byproduct later, but leaving them with your marijuana can lower the quality and give your bud a harsher taste.

Take the buds and use a string or another system to hang them in a cool, dark place that is relatively dry. You will want them to dry until you can easily snap the buds off the stem when you apply pressure. If they are not ready, they will only bend.

Curing Your Buds

Once you have dried your marijuana buds, you are still not ready to smoke if you want the highest quality. The key to high quality is getting the perfect balance of stickiness, without the marijuana getting too dry. Remove the excess stem from your buds and place them in a mason jar or another airtight container. Place them in a cool, dark area for at least 2 weeks, but no longer than one month. Open the container at least once per day, being sure that any moisture in the container is released. Moisture can cause mold growth and ruin your entire harvest, so use caution and be sure that buds are dried thoroughly before you attempt curing them.

Conclusion: Step 6-Enjoy!

Congratulations! If you have reached this point in the book, then you are probably a marijuana growing expert!

The next logical step is to put your skills to the test, if you have not jumped in and gotten your hands dirty already. It is important to remember that there is more than one successful method for growing cannabis and only you can decide what is the best option for you. Whether you want to grow inside or outside, there is more than one technique you can choose. Additionally, each method has its own advantages and disadvantages, as well as costs to consider before you get started.

Remember that growing marijuana is a process. The more that you put your skills to the test, the more you will learn about taking care of your plants. You will find your own preferred balance of water, lighting, and nutrients to help each harvest grow bigger and better than your last. Additionally, don't be afraid to switch up your techniques as you grow your marijuana operation!

Best of luck for a successful harvest!

Made in the USA
San Bernardino, CA
22 April 2018